Interferon 7

Interferon 7

1986

ION GRESSER
Editor-in-chief

1986

ACADEMIC PRESS
Harcourt Brace Jovanovich, Publishers
London Orlando San Diego New York Austin
Boston Toronto Sydney Tokyo

ACADEMIC PRESS INC. (LONDON) LTD.
24/28 Oval Road
London NW1

United States Edition published by
ACADEMIC PRESS INC.
Orlando, Florida 32887

British Library Cataloguing in Publication Data

Interferon 7.
1. Interferon
I. Gresser, Ion
616.07'9 QR187.5

ISBN 0-12-302256-8

Printed in Great Britain at the Alden Press, Oxford

Contributors

Danièle Brouty-Boyé, *Laboratory of Viral Oncology, Institut de Recherches Scientifiques sur le Cancer, Boîte Postale No 8, 94802 Villejuif France*

R. Camble, *ICI Pharmaceuticals Division, Alderley Park, Macclesfield, SK10 4TG, UK*

F. J. Carr, *ICI Pharmaceuticals Division, Alderley Park, Macclesfield, SK10 4TG, UK*

Madeleine M. Cochet, *Biologie Moléculaire du Gène, Unité INSERM 277, Institut Pasteur, 25 rue du Docteur Roux, 75724 Paris Cedex 15, France*

M. D. Edge, *ICI Pharmaceuticals Division, Alderley Park, Macclesfield, SK10 4TG, UK*

Marc Fellous, *Immunogénétique Humaine, Unité INSERM 276, Institut Pasteur, 25 rue du Docteur Roux, 75724 Paris Cedex 15, France*

J. E. Fitton, *ICI Pharmaceuticals Division, Alderley Park, Macclesfield, SK10 4TG, UK*

R. C. Hockney, *ICI Pharmaceuticals Division, Alderley Park, Macclesfield, SK10 4TG, UK*

Gerald J. Jonak, *E.I. du Pont de Nemours & Co Inc, Central Research and Development Department, Wilmington, DE 19898, USA*

Ernest Knight Jnr, *E.I. du Pont de Nemours & Co Inc, Central Research and Development Department, Wilmington, DE 19898, USA*

Susan E. Krown, *Clinical Immunology Service, Department of Medicine, Memorial Sloan-Kettering Cancer Center, New York, NY 10021, USA*

V. E. Moore, *ICI Pharmaceuticals Division, Alderley Park, Macclesfield, SK10 4TG, UK*

Carl F. Nathan, *Laboratory of Cellular Physiology and Immunology, The Rockefeller University, New York, NY 10021, USA* (Present address: *Division of Hematology-Oncology, Department of Medicine, Cornell University Medical College, 1300 York Avenue, New York, NY 10021, USA*)

Frédéric M. Rosa, *Immunogénétique Humaine, Unité INSERM 276, Institut Pasteur, 25 rue du Docteur Roux, 75724 Paris Cedex 15, France*

David Wallach, *Department of Virology, The Weizmann Institute of Science, Rehovot, Israel*

Contents

Cytotoxins (Tumour Necrosis Factor, Lymphotoxin and Others): Molecular and Functional Characteristics and Interactions with Interferons

David Wallach

Peroxide and Pteridine: A Hypothesis on the Regulation of Macrophage Antimicrobial Activity by Interferon γ

Carl F. Nathan

Interferon and the Tumour Cell Phenotype

Danièle Brouty-Boyé

Interferons and the Regulation of Oncogenes

Gerald J. Jonak and Ernest Knight, Jr

AIDS and Kaposi's Sarcoma: Interferons in Pathogenesis and Treatment

Susan E. Krown

Interferon Analogues from Synthetic Genes: An Approach to Protein Structure–Activity Studies

M. D. EDGE, R. CAMBLE, V. E. MOORE, R. C. HOCKNEY, F. J. CARR AND J. E. FITTON

ICI Pharmaceuticals Division, Alderley Park, Macclesfield, Cheshire SK10 4TG, U.K.

INTERFERON 7
ISBN 0 12 302256 8

I INTRODUCTION

In the search for better medicines, the study of structure–activity relationships in a lead drug to find analogues with improved therapeutic properties requires close collaboration between chemists and bioscientists. With low-molecular-weight compounds, the medicinal chemist normally assumes responsibility for all phases of analogue design, synthesis, purification and characterization. This simple situation no longer applies when the starting structure is a protein, and the approach to analogue production lies through recombinant DNA technology. The disparate skills of protein scientists, nucleotide chemists, molecular biologists and microbiologists must all be integrated to fulfil the role traditionally played by the medicinal chemist. To succeed, a high level of mutual appreciation must be built up of the contribution and challenges demanded of each discipline.

Thus, when the first two authors were invited to review our experiences with the preparation and biological evaluation of interferon analogues from synthetic genes, it was natural to involve other senior collaborators in this account of what was a shared personal experience. We have indulged fully in the freedom provided by this review series to concentrate on our own work in the hope of leaving the reader with a better impression of the considerations, both practical and conceptual, that contribute to the strategies adopted and the excitement generated in multidisciplinary projects of this kind.

II BACKGROUND

The events that led to our interest in interferon analogues can be traced back to April 1980. We had recently established novel procedures for solid-phase synthesis of oligonucleotides (Gait *et al.*, 1980), required mainly as probes and primers by molecular biologists. Until that time, gene synthesis techniques had been limited to the construction of relatively small genes because solution-phase methodology for oligonucleotide synthesis was a time-consuming process. We were therefore eager to apply our new synthetic procedures to the assembly of a much larger gene. We set ourselves the task of synthesizing and cloning a gene for human IFN-α_1 (Edge *et al.*, 1981). Expression of this gene first from a *lac* UV5 promoter (De Maeyer *et al.*, 1982) and later from a synthetic *trp* promoter (Windass *et al.*, 1982) gave us the encouragement to embark on a programme of work to explore structure–function relationships of such a large protein.

By the time expression of IFN-α_1 from our synthetic IFN gene had been demonstrated (which was less than 12 months from the start of the work), it was clear that several IFN-α genes existed (Nagata *et al.*, 1980; Goeddel *et al.*, 1981) and that IFN-α_2 was 50 times more active than IFN-α_1 on human cells. It also seemed likely that IFN-α_2 (or IFN-αA) would be the first recombinant interferon to enter clinical studies. For these reasons we decided to base our structure–function programme on IFN-α_2. This required synthesis of another gene for the new parent protein (Edge *et al.*, 1983); however, it did allow us to incorporate certain improvements to the synthetic technology and purification procedures. A modified ligation strategy also took into account the long-term nature of the programme and provision was made for quantitation and storage of intermediate double-stranded DNA fragments.

The synthetic IFN-α_2 gene gave very poor expression from the *lac* UV5 promoter but adequate levels of the protein were obtained when the gene was placed downstream from a synthetic *trp* promoter. The electrophoretic and biological properties of the expressed product were indistinguishable from authentic interferon α_2.

III OBJECTIVES

The desire to create novel analogues of naturally occurring proteins to understand better the structural basis of their biological functions is not new. Ultimately such knowledge could lead to the design of products with improved profiles of activity or stability for clinical and industrial use. Over many years protein chemists have approached the problem by chemical derivatization of natural proteins, by protein semisynthesis (fragmentation of native protein followed by re-assembly with one fragment replaced by a synthetic peptide incorporating the desired structural modification), and even by the complete chemical synthesis of proteins. However, even when successful, such techniques are limited either by the availability of the native protein or by the time, effort and cost involved. Following the dramatic success of recombinant DNA technology in providing an abundant supply of native proteins, several techniques have been devised to construct new genes that direct the synthesis of novel protein analogues. In the last 4 years, hybrid gene formation, site-directed mutagenesis and total gene synthesis have all been applied by different groups to produce interferon analogues (for a review of such work with interferon see Edge and Camble, 1984).

Hybrid genes, by definition, are able to provide only novel combinations of the amino acid residues that occur naturally in the parent protein sequences. They cannot produce changes at amino acid positions conserved between the parents or substitute completely different amino acids at non-conserved positions. Site-directed mutagenesis was still being developed when we began our study and was only being used to create gene deletions or change amino acid residues one or two at a time. We focused on exploiting our synthetic gene expertise and assessing its ability to generate interferon analogues for structure–activity studies. Synthetic genes offer an extremely versatile approach whereby, in principle, any genetically coded amino acid residue can be placed at any number of positions anywhere along the entire length of the polypeptide chain.

We set out to explore three broad objectives:

1. *Can analogues be produced at a reasonable rate?* The ability of recombinant DNA techniques to provide protein analogues, coupled with hopes that computer modelling will facilitate prediction of the effects of structural changes in proteins on their functions, has created much excitement about the ease of "protein engineering". In our view, a substantial number of analogues covering a range of structural variants will have to be examined before any therapeutically significant change in biological profile can be expected.

This is certainly still the experience in most small-molecule medicinal chemistry and there is no convincing reason why the problem should be easier for a complex protein structure. Such philosophy implies that the ability to produce interferon analogues is not enough. To be of real use, the technology must also permit a good throughput of analogues. We felt that the equivalent of about one new analogue a week was a necessary goal to work towards.

2. *Do the products give coherent structure–function profiles?* If gene synthesis, cloning and expression could achieve the hoped-for level of productivity, it would not be possible to carry out rigorous purification and detailed structural analysis of every interferon analogue protein. Knowing the coding gene sequence for the analogues to be correct, we hoped that protein extracts would provide consistent target protein sequence–activity patterns, when purified only to a stage at which bacterial contaminants do not interfere in the assays. Only analogues with profiles of interest would be characterized in detail.

3. *Can the different biological activities of IFN-α_2 be separated?* Series of analogues can be used to address many questions of scientific interest, but the ultimate medicinal chemical justification for the study of structure–activity relationships is to provide an improved therapeutic agent. IFN-α_2 has well-defined antiviral, antiproliferative and immuno-modulating activities. An analogue with increased selectivity between these activities might alleviate some of the side-effects observed clinically with purified natural IFN and recombinant IFN-α_2. Increased selectivity of action was also an objective that could be assessed by comparing ratios of titres in the different assays.

This is possible using partially purified extracts and does not demand measurement of absolute potencies, which requires pure products.

IV TYPES OF ANALOGUES EXAMINED

Target analogues were selected to reflect several different themes:

1. Truncations
2. IFN-α_2/α_1 hybrids
3. IFN-α_2/γ hybrids
4. Replacement of residues of a specific amino acid
5. Changes at the Cys29-Cys138 disulphide bridge
6. Clusters of conserved amino acids.

As well as probing structure–activity relationships, these were designed to test the gene synthesis and cloning methodology, and to provide some idea of how great a change might be introduced before compromising the stability of the interferon protein in *Escherichia coli*.

V TECHNOLOGY OF ANALOGUE PRODUCTION

This section presents the chemical and biochemical techniques we have used and how they have been integrated to produce interferon analogues from synthetic genes. The major steps are summarized in Fig. 1.

A Synthesis of Oligonucleotides

The rapid synthesis of genes involves enzymic ligation of a series of short overlapping complementary oligonucleotides (usually containing 10–20 nucleotide units). Nearly 70 such oligonucleotides are required for a gene encoding an interferon and more than 12 alternative oligonucleotides may be needed to construct a gene for each analogue. The ability, therefore, to rapidly synthesize oligonucleotides of defined length and sequence is a prerequisite for any structure–function programme with proteins obtained by bacterial expression of cloned synthetic genes.

Oligonucleotide synthesis has developed over the past decade from a slow and laborious process requiring expertise and specialist knowledge to a rapid, routine procedure which can be readily automated. For many years, the basic procedure used by specialist groups has been the improved phosphotriester method. When used for synthesis in solution, this method requires the chromatographic purification of each protected intermediate during construction of each oligonucleotide sequence. The development of a

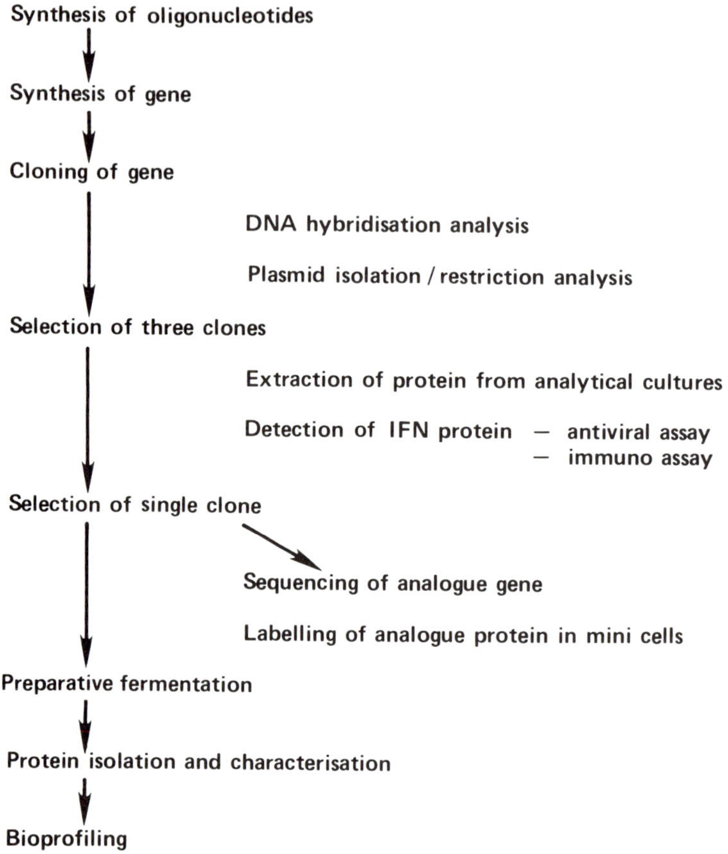

Fig. 1 Outline scheme for analogue production and evaluation.

reliable solid-phase phosphotriester approach avoided the need for repeated chromatographic purification of intermediates and increased the rate of synthesis by an order of magnitude. Although a variety of solid supports has been successfully employed for oligonucleotide synthesis, we used a polydimethylacrylamide resin developed at the MRC laboratory in Cambridge by Drs Bob Sheppard and Mike Gait (Gait and Sheppard, 1977). A summary of the basic procedure is presented in Fig. 2.

A mononucleotide attached to the support is partially deprotected by treatment with acid. Further blocks of dinucleotides (or mononucleotides) are added in a stepwise manner using a coupling reagent such as MSNT until

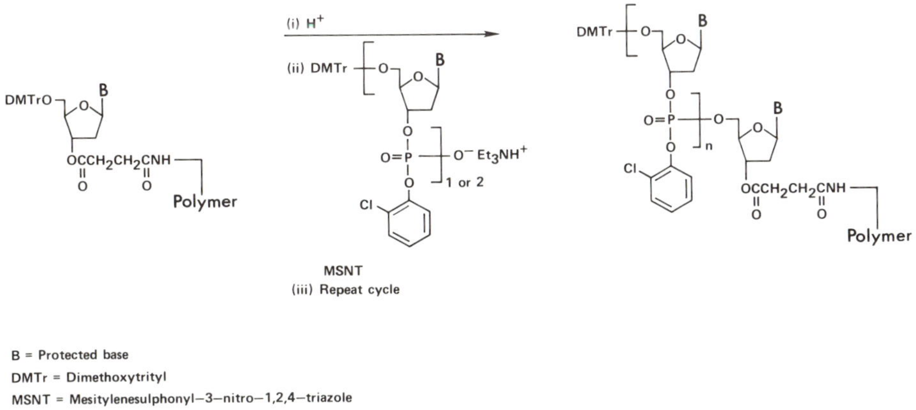

Fig. 2 Outline scheme for solid-phase synthesis of oligonucleotides.

the desired sequence of bases has been assembled. The deprotection and washing steps are carried out by a simple filtration procedure. All protecting groups are removed from the final sequence and the oligonucleotide is purified by high-performance liquid chromatography (HPLC), initially using ion-exchange on Partisil 10-SAX. Further purification is achieved by reverse-phase HPLC on a μ-Bondapak C_{18} column.

Using such methodologies, together with a semi-automated solvent delivery system, the oligonucleotides used in the IFN-α_1 gene synthesis were prepared at the rate of 1 to 2 per day. Starting from 100 mg of functionalized resin, several OD_{260} units of purified oligonucleotides were often prepared. Certain sequences, however, proved difficult to purify owing to irreversible adsorption of the product on the HPLC column matrix (Markham *et al.*, 1980). This led us to develop an improved elution buffer, containing formamide, for ion-exchange HPLC (Newton *et al.*, 1983). For the IFN-α_2 gene synthesis, several minor technical changes had improved the rate of synthesis and yields of oligonucleotides. These changes, together with our improved HPLC procedure permitted oligonucleotide preparation on half the earlier scale. This significantly reduced the demand for intermediate monomers and dimers and would have allowed us to synthesize oligonucleotides sufficiently rapidly to carry out an interferon analogue programme. However, another major development, this time in the support used for oligonucleotide synthesis, made the whole procedure even more efficient. The introduction of rigid solid supports, based on controlled-pore glass or a Keiselguhr-polydimethylacrylamide composite resin, enabled syntheses to be performed in small glass columns with a flow-through system for the washing steps (Gait *et al.*, 1982). This increased the ease with which several syntheses could be performed simultaneously.

Improvements in oligonucleotide chemistry are still being made. Reaction times have been reduced by the use of catalysts or elevated temperatures and better protecting groups are being developed. Several reliable automated DNA synthesizers are now commercially available and a manual method for the simultaneous synthesis of large numbers of oligonucleotides, the segmental disc approach (Frank *et al.*, 1983), has been developed. Clearly, the availability of oligonucleotides is no longer a limiting factor for assembly of synthetic genes.

B Synthesis of Genes

In this review, gene synthesis refers to the assembly of synthetic oligonucleotides into double-stranded DNA encoding an interferon. Two major steps are involved in going from oligonucleotides to double-stranded DNA fragments. Firstly, the 5′-hydroxyl group is phosphorylated with [γ-^{32}P]ATP using polynucleotide kinase. The radioactive label introduced by this reaction enables small quantities of oligonucleotides and DNA fragments to be detected on gels by autoradiography. The second step involves spontaneous alignment of groups of phosphorylated oligonucleotides (to form a double-stranded complex by an annealing process) and joining of adjacent oligonucleotides in each strand using T4 DNA ligase.

For assembly of the 68 oligonucleotides comprising the IFN-α_2 gene sequence (and most analogues), twelve groups of 5 and one group of 8 oligonucleotides were initially ligated (Fig. 3). In anticipation that these small DNA sub-fragments (A to M in Fig. 3) would also serve as intermediates for analogue gene production, the 5′-protruding end of each double-stranded product was left unphosphorylated. They were quantified using the low-specific-activity internal labels. At a later date, when the internal labels had decayed, this allowed aliquots to be freshly labelled at the 5′ end immediately before use for gene assembly. Following the strategy outlined in Fig. 3 the small sub-fragments A to M were sequentially ligated to give the large sub-fragments I to III and then the final gene. For our IFN-α_2 gene, the first pair of oligonucleotides was designed for expression from a *lac* UV5 promoter. For convenient synthesis of analogue genes these were replaced by sequences that could be joined directly to our synthetic *trp* promoter.

The starting point for IFN-α_2 analogue genes was resynthesis of appropriate oligonucleotides encoding the proposed changes in amino acid sequence. For a single amino acid alteration, two new oligonucleotides were synthesized, or three if the amino acid codon occurred at a ligation point in

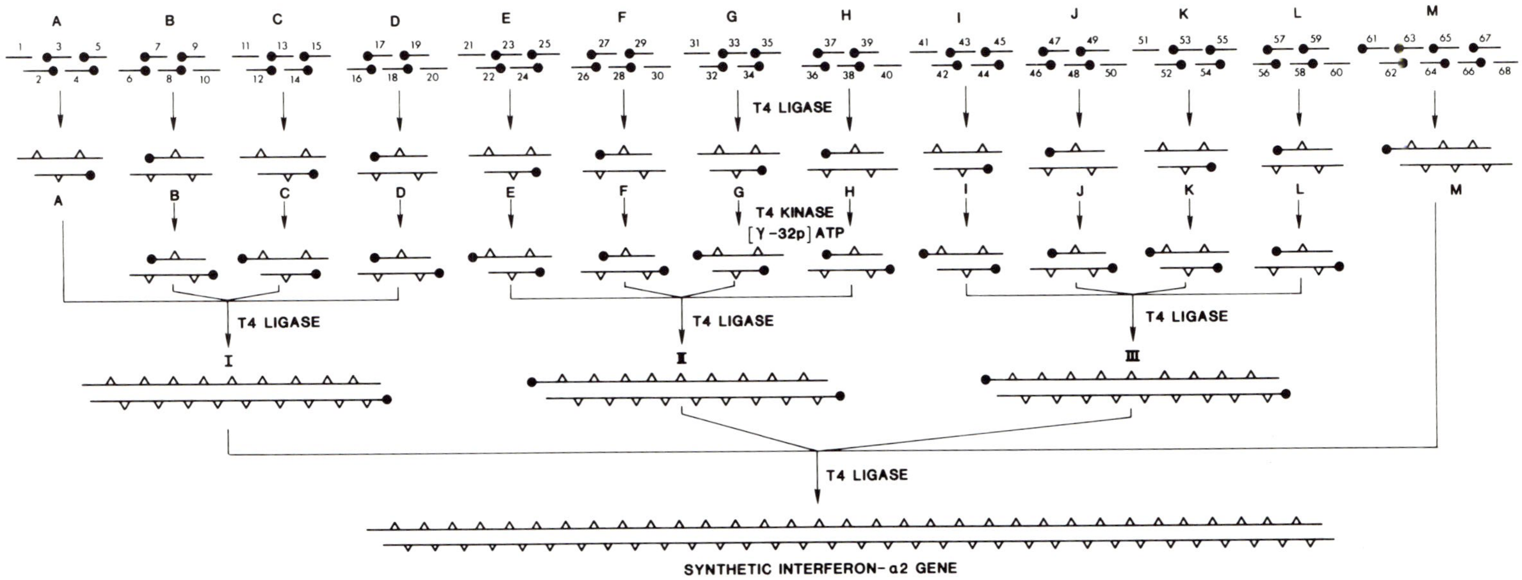

Fig. 3 Scheme of the ligation of chemically synthesized oligonucleotides (1 to 68) to construct a gene for IFN-α_2 (Edge *et al.*, 1983). Aliquots of the oligonucleotides, except 1, 10, 11, 20, 21, 30, 31, 40, 41, 50, 51, 60 and 68 were phosphorylated with T4-induced polynucleotide kinase and [γ^{32}P]ATP. The terminal phosphate group is represented by the dot. Thirteen separate T4 ligase-catalysed joining reactions were performed to generate small sub-fragments A to M. Large subfragments I to III were constructed from fragments A to L after phosphorylation of fragments B to L. For most analogue gene constructs, fragment III included fragment M. The final ligation of I to III plus M (or I to III if M was already included) gave the complete gene.

the DNA sequence. Since any genetically coded amino acid residue can be substituted, added or deleted at any position throughout the polypeptide chain, synthetic genes are particularly attractive for introducing multiple changes. Thus, for example, to produce five simultaneous changes at widely spaced positions, a maximum of 15 new oligonucleotides are required.

With the ligation strategy shown in Fig. 3 these new oligonucleotides were substituted for the original sequences. No allowance was made for potential secondary structure formation, but we accepted that preparation of some DNA fragments might give problems. For the annealing step prior to ligation, an aqueous solution of the oligonucleotide mixture was heated to 100°C and either slowly cooled to room temperature (over ~6 hours) or rapidly cooled by immersion in an ice bath. If neither protocol resulted in formation of the expected DNA strands after ligation, the problem was usually circumvented by leaving out one oligonucleotide in an initial reaction, then joining it to the duplex in a second step.

Assembly of the small DNA sub-fragments into analogue genes followed a pattern similar to that described for the parent gene (Fig. 3), but the final small sub-fragment (Group M) was incorporated into fragment III. Yields of the synthetic genes varied considerably and at least three contributory factors have been identified. Firstly, on extended storage, some small DNA sub-fragments themselves adsorbed on to the walls of the storage container which invalidated the initial quantitation. Even small errors in the stoichiometry of the multiple sub-fragments used in ligation reactions resulted in drastic reduction of product yields. A second problem involved the polynucleotide kinase enzyme which is used to phosphorylate the DNA fragments prior to ligation. We found that this enzyme activity must be completely removed from the reaction mixture before the ligation step to avoid formation of high-MW impurities that reduced yields and complicated identification of the desired product. A simple freeze–thaw method was inadequate and extraction with phenol/chloroform was required. Finally, and most importantly, erratic adsorption of ligation product during purification by polyacrylamide gel electrophoresis was a problem. This could be largely avoided by ensuring complete removal of protein from the sample before loading on the gel and by the use of freshly prepared acrylamide solution for gel formation.

Once a discrete region of the molecule had been identified for more detailed structure–function studies, the efficiency of analogue production could be significantly improved by generating a vector already containing most of the remainder of the IFN gene sequence. For example, the unique *Bst*EII restriction site at the codons for amino acid residues 44 to 46 was exploited to produce a vector containing the IFN-α_2 gene sequence encoding amino acids 46 to 165. With this vector, changes within the first 43 amino acids were accomplished by preparing synthetic fragments spanning only the first 45 amino acids. Only one ligation step was necessary to produce these small fragments (about one-third of the complete gene), which could be purified by gel electrophoresis to give amounts adequate for cloning.

As an extension of this approach, we prepared an IFN-α_2 gene containing several unique restriction sites. This has been used to generate a series of plasmid vectors encoding large sections of the IFN-α_2 gene sequence for rapid analogue production.

C Cloning and Characterization of Genes

1 *Cloning of complete genes*

The multiple-stage procedure used originally for expression of our synthetic IFN-α_2 gene under *trp* promoter control (Edge *et al.*, 1983) was clearly unsuitable for routine preparation of analogues. Thus we redesigned the gene to allow direct cloning into plasmid pSTPI (Fig. 4). This plasmid has a synthetic *trp* promoter ending in a unique *Cla*I restriction site (Windass *et al.*, 1982). Genes flanked by *Taq*I (which has the same cohesive end as *Cla*I) and *Sal*I restriction sites and containing an initiation codon just downstream from the *Taq*I site were expressed when cloned in this vector. The system was first tested using a new gene for IFN-α_2 that was readily cloned and gave a level of expression similar to the original construction.

To avoid losses associated with gel purification of the small quantities (5–200 fmole) of synthetic genes, the final ligation mixtures, still containing large sub-fragments (I to III, Fig. 3), were used directly for cloning. A 2 : 1 ratio of vector to synthetic DNA termini was found to be optimal in yielding recombinants. *E. coli* strain JA221 was the usual host organism, although MM294 has also been used; a new transformation procedure (Hanahan, 1983) improved the efficiency of cloning. Recombinants containing analogue genes were identified as tetracycline-sensitive colonies among a background of tetracycline-resistant colonies harbouring the reformed parent plasmid (pSTPI). When we were attempting to clone very small amounts of synthetic genes, this background could account for the majority of transformants despite careful purification of the *Cla*I-*Sal*I vector fragment. Tetracycline-sensitive transformants were subjected to colony hybridization analysis with small sub-group fragments (30/45 mers) labelled with ^{32}P by nick translation. Candidate analogue gene recombinants were screened with two probes, one homologous to a common IFN-α_2 region and the other homologous to an analogue specific DNA sequence. DNA was prepared from hybridization-positive clones and subjected to restriction analysis with *Hpa*II endonuclease to confirm the expected DNA fragment pattern.

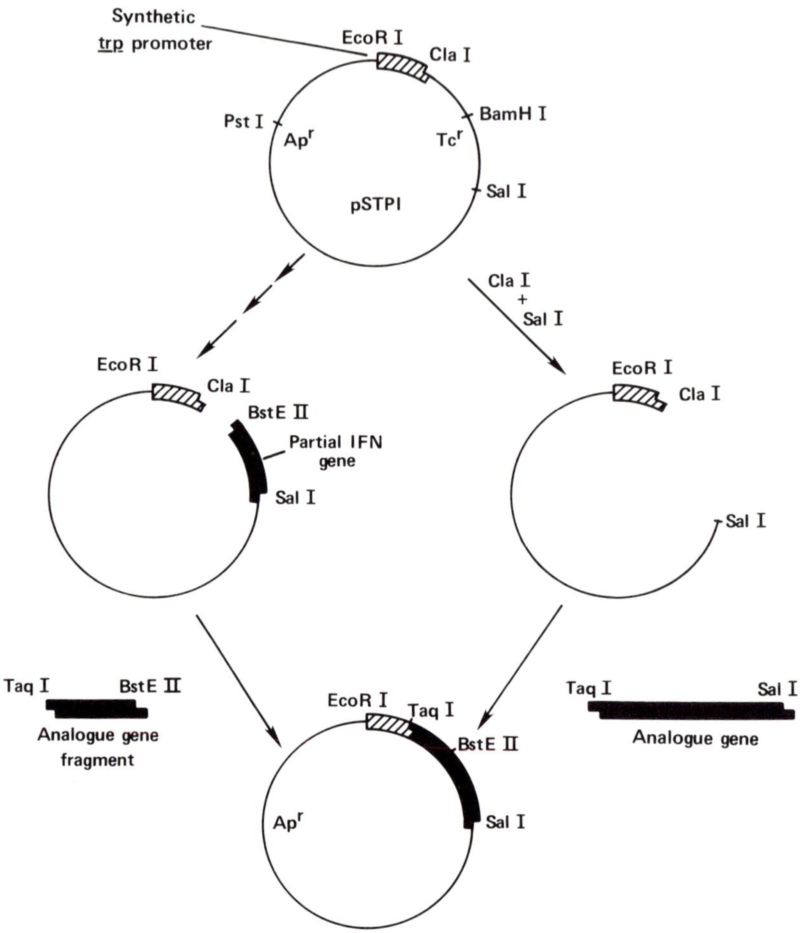

Fig. 4 Schematic representation of the construction of recombinant plasmids containing IFN analogue genes under *trp* promoter control.

2 Cloning of gene fragments

As described in section V (B), synthetic gene fragments were used to prepare analogues with changes only within the first 45 amino acid residues. The analogue genes so produced, however, are under the same transcriptional and translational control as the complete genes. Unlike the situation with pSTPI, where background colonies were easily identified by their tetracycline resistance, the vector used to clone these gene fragments was derived from an IFN-α_2 expression plasmid (pIFS1205) and gave tetracycline-sensitive background colonies that also contained the parent IFN-α_2 gene. Recombinants containing the desired analogue gene could only be distinguished using ^{32}P-labelled oligonucleotide probes corresponding to analogue specific sequences. Screening conditions could be adjusted to detect changes in a single base pair; however, for each different gene this involved a laborious series of washes at different specific temperatures. An alternative strategy was therefore developed to eliminate this background of colonies expressing IFN-α_2. The *Taq*I-*Bst*EII IFN-α_2 gene fragment in the parental cloning vector was replaced with a 1.3 kb *Cla*I-*Bst*EII "stuffer" DNA fragment from phage λ. This allowed colonies containing analogue genes to be distinguished by screening with small sub-fragment probes from the *Taq*I-*Bst*EII region of the IFN-α_2 gene. DNA was then prepared from three clones and subjected to restriction analysis as described for the complete genes.

3 *Characterization of cloned genes*

Cell lysates from 100-ml cultures of up to three selected clones (*E. coli* strains JA221 or DS410) were tested for IFN-like activity in antiviral and NK2-monoclonal antibody immunoradiometric (NK2-IRMA) assays. In the absence of either activity, the presence of any new protein was detected by fluorography after PAGE-SDS of plasmid-encoded proteins labelled in *E. coli* minicells (Streuli *et al.*, 1981). This also provided the first indication of the molecular size and quality of expressed analogue protein. Although we hoped for consistency within the three selected clones, we found some variability which could have arisen from false positives in the hybridization procedure or from mutational events arising during gene synthesis or cloning. From the accumulated data a single clone was selected for each analogue and plasmid DNA isolated for DNA sequence determination.

It was not practicable routinely to sequence the gene from more than one clone for each analogue. Generating sequence data for even one clone per analogue proved time-consuming, especially when every base had to be confirmed, and was usually a retrospective process. Initially we concentrated on confirming the sequence of the changed regions by the use of the dideoxy chain termination method performed on linearized plasmid DNA (Wallace *et al.*, 1981). Later, the *trp* promoter–analogue gene fragment was cloned into M13 vectors and most of the gene sequence was established for each analogue. Genes were fully characterized for all analogues with unusual profiles of activity. Occasionally the selected clone was found to contain the parent IFN-α_2 gene or an unplanned gene mutation. A small number of analogue genes gave regions of equivocal sequence and some work is still in progress to establish the true sequence. In retrospect it would have been prudent not to limit ourselves to a detailed examination of only a single clone. On a few occasions, a desired analogue was not obtained simply because the selected clone was shown to be wrong after gene sequencing.

D Preparative Fermentation of Recombinant Bacteria

The selected clone harbouring each analogue gene in the tryptophan auxotrophic *E. coli* strain JA221 was grown in 4×1l shake-flask batches in minimal medium containing a low concentration of tryptophan (2 μg/ml) essentially as described for IFN-α_1 (Windass *et al.*, 1982). This provided tryptophan-limited growth to an OD of 1.0 and the accumulated interferons were released in soluble form following lysis of bacteria by lysozyme treatment and sonication. This system gave about 10^7 NK2-IRMA U/l/OD ($\sim 5\,\mu$g) of most analogue proteins in the lysate supernatant, which was sufficient for structure–function studies but somewhat lower than had been achieved with IFN-α_2 (Edge *et al.*, 1983).

Later, we found *E. coli* strain DS410 accumulated 20-fold higher levels of IFN-α_2. Furthermore, this strain is prototrophic and grows in our routine medium to an OD of ~ 3. By adopting DS410 as the preferred host strain for interferon analogue expression, the volume of culture required was reduced to 900 ml. Unfortunately only 2 analogues accumulated to the same level as IFN-α_2 in DS410; most achieved only the same levels as with JA221. Differential stability of the expressed proteins is the most likely explanation of these observations, but there is no obvious relationship between analogue sequence and such assumed lability. In the future it may be advantageous to use protease-deficient host strains for expression of analogue proteins.

At the outset, most IFN-α_2 activity was recovered in soluble form in supernatants following lysozyme lysis. Over time, variable amounts of IFN-α_2 were associated with the insoluble pellet fraction from both JA221 and DS410. Product could be solubilized by extraction with SDS or guanidine-HCl. This same phenomenon also occurred with analogues. The low titres in supernatants from non-detergent lyses were undesirable for structure–activity studies as they introduce the possibility that the material may in some way be unrepresentative of the bulk of the expressed product. The solubility and physical state of heterologous proteins expressed in *E. coli* are affected by fermentation conditions in a poorly understood manner and, especially for structure–function studies, it is essential that all possible steps be taken to ensure constancy of all growth and processing routines.

E Isolation of IFN Analogues for Assay

From our own experience and that quoted in the literature with IFN-α_1 and IFN-α_2 we anticipated that the IFN analogue products would represent less than 0.1% of the total protein produced by the bacteria, and would be present largely in soluble form in the supernatant fractions from *E. coli* lysates. In these quantities, IFN protein is not detectable on PAGE-SDS gels against the background of *E. coli* proteins. Trial studies with IFN-α_1, IFN-α_2 and control bacterial extracts indicated that lysate supernatants, and re-extracted protein precipitates therefrom, were not suitable for all bioprofiling assays. A further routine chromatography step was needed before biological evaluation.

Adsorption chromatographic procedures were unattractive, as analogues could be expected to show varying elution characteristics and it would be necessary to assay across eluate fractions each time to identify those containing the product. This was not just a theoretical concern, for we had already discovered that, whereas IFN-α_2 was retained by Blue Sepharose and NK2-Sepharose, IFN-α_1 not only did not elute in a similar fashion but actually passed unretarded through columns of both supports.*

Fortunately, size exclusion chromatography on Ultragel AcA54 of protein extracts from *E. coli* lysate supernatants separated over 80% of bacterial protein from the IFN products. Analogues were recovered with confidence by collecting a rather broad fraction around the elution position of IFN-α_1 and IFN-α_2. The analogue products were still less than 1% pure, but the remaining bacterial contaminants did not interfere in the biological assays. This was confirmed later by showing that, for almost all analogues, samples prepared in this way and samples purified by monoclonal antibody affinity chromatography gave very similar ratios between titres in the human antiviral, antiproliferative and NK-cell stimulating bioassays and the NK2-immunoradiometric assay used for profiling.

This gel filtration procedure was used routinely for almost a year to prepare samples of some fifty different analogues for initial structure–activity studies. One problem was contamination of an analogue with 0.01–0.1% of the preceding analogue purified on the same column (demonstrated by running an antiviral active or NK2-cross-reactive analogue followed by an inactive analogue). Such levels of cross-contamination would not seriously mask a good separation of activities in an active analogue, but they do produce significant titres in an analogue that is really inactive. Since it is uneconomic to provide a new column for each analogue, we used one column for antiviral active analogues (shown by assay of initial lysate supernatants) and a second column for antiviral inactive analogues.

* This differential behaviour of IFN-α_2 and IFN-α_1 on Blue Sepharose is of general interest, being consistent with a report (Traub *et al.*, 1981) that human lymphoblastoid (Namalva) IFN can be separated into bound and unretained fractions on this support. The bound fraction, like IFN-α_2, was reported to be about equi-active on human and bovine cells; the unretained fraction, like IFN-α_1, was much more active on bovine cells than on human cells.

A limitation we had accepted with this approach to analogue screening was an absence of any information on the homogeneity of the analogue-related protein present in the samples being profiled. Our only indication of the quality of the protein products came from the minicell radio-labelling experiments described earlier. We were very conscious that a correct analogue gene sequence is a requisite but not a guarantee of a correct monocomponent analogue protein product. Changes programmed into the gene may indicate only the minimal structural difference of the protein product from the parent IFN-α_2. As described in more detail below, we have detected heterogeneities arising from retention of variable amounts of *N*-terminal initiator methionine residue, from monomer species with incomplete or incorrect disulphide bridge formation, from oligomer species linked in most cases through intermolecular disulphides and from truncated species probably produced by bacterial protease activity. In spite of these uncertainties, comparison of activity profiles between samples of different analogues prepared in this way provided remarkably coherent patterns of target sequence–activity data.

About a year into the programme we wanted to measure the effects of analogues on release of interleukin-1. Since the assay involved was sensitive to bacterial endotoxin, the products obtained by gel filtration were no longer adequate. Experience with the first 50 analogue sequences suggested that the majority of structural variants should be recognized by either the NK2 or the more recently available YOK monoclonal antibody reagents (Celltech Ltd, Slough, U.K.). Therefore, a new routine was developed in which crude lysate supernatants of all analogues, old and new, were purified by immunoaffinity chromatography on NK2- or YOK-Sepharose. A separate column was used for each analogue avoiding any risk of cross-contamination. A single run on 200 μl bed volume of support yielded 10–50 μg of analogue protein. This was enough for all the assays and also allowed the quality of samples, which now contained only target analogue-related protein, to be monitored by PAGE-SDS using a sensitive silver staining procedure. In many instances it was also possible to produce gels stained with Coomassie blue from which estimates of protein content were obtained using a scanning densitometer, allowing us to convert titres into specific activities.

VI QUALITY OF PROTEIN PRODUCTS

The availability of immobilized monoclonal antibody facilitates the rapid isolation of interferon analogue proteins and ensures that the purified products are immunologically related to the parent molecule. However, these products may still be a mixture of protein species and any analogues of special interest should be further characterized using a broad range of physico-chemical techniques. Each of the following analytical methods has been used within the IFN programme.

A SDS Polyacrylamide Gel Electrophoresis (PAGE-SDS)

This technique has remained our basic analytical procedure for confirming the molecular weight and gross purity of immunoaffinity-purified recombinant proteins, and has proved to be particularly useful for the detection of proteolytic degradation products and for *N*- and *C*-terminally truncated analogues. PAGE-SDS in the absence of reductant gives some indication of the redox status and the degree of intermolecular disulphide bond formation in the interferon proteins. Oligomer formation was observed most frequently in analogues containing odd numbers of cysteine residues.

B Immunoblotting

We have raised polyclonal antisera against purified recombinant IFN-α_2 as immunogen. These have been particularly useful when used for immunoblotting of PAGE-SDS gels (Towbin and Gordon, 1984) to detect those few analogues that failed to cross-react with either NK2 or YOK monoclonal antibody.

C Amino Acid Composition Analysis

Amino acid composition analysis with the traditional ninhydrin detection procedure has been used to confirm the presence of programmed changes in selected analogues. Recently we have been investigating the new PICO-TAG (Millipore, Waters Chromatography Division) procedure, which utilizes pre-column derivatization with phenyl isothiocyanate (Bidlingmeyer *et al.*, 1984). Results indicate that the greatly increased sensitivity of this HPLC-based system will be extremely useful for compositional comparisons of analogue proteins only available in limited quantities.

D *N*-terminal Sequence Analysis

Automated *N*-terminal sequence determinations have confirmed the presence of programmed changes in a few selected analogues with altered amino acid residues within approximately 35 residues of the protein *N*-terminus (e.g. [Ala^{30,32,33}]IFN-α_2 and [Leu^{16,21,59,111,148}]IFN-α_2). *N*-terminal sequencing should be particularly useful for *N*-terminally-truncated analogues and for identifying analogues proteolytically degraded at the *N*-terminus. It also indicates partial retention, in analogues, of *N*-terminal initiator methionine residue, which has been reported to be partially removed from recombinant IFN-α_2 expressed in *E. coli* (Wetzel *et al.*, 1981).

E HPLC Analysis

Reverse-phase HPLC is a major method for protein characterization offering speed, sensitivity and high resolution and is complementary to PAGE-SDS. Reverse-phase chromatography of immunoaffinity-purified IFN-α_2 and analogues exhibiting minimal heterogeneity on PAGE-SDS has, in several cases, indicated that the products are heterogeneous. The relative amounts of the multiple components vary from one preparation to another. We believe this reflects the disulphide bonding pattern and general redox status of the isolated proteins.

Figure 5a shows a typical reverse-phase HPLC pattern given by IFN-α_2 after purification on NK2-Sepharose. Peaks 1 and 2 probably correspond to the "fast" and "slow" interferon monomers identified on non-reducing PAGE-SDS gels (Felix *et al.*, 1985) and are thought to consist of correctly disulphide-bonded and partially-reduced IFN (Cysl and 98 free SH) respectively. The

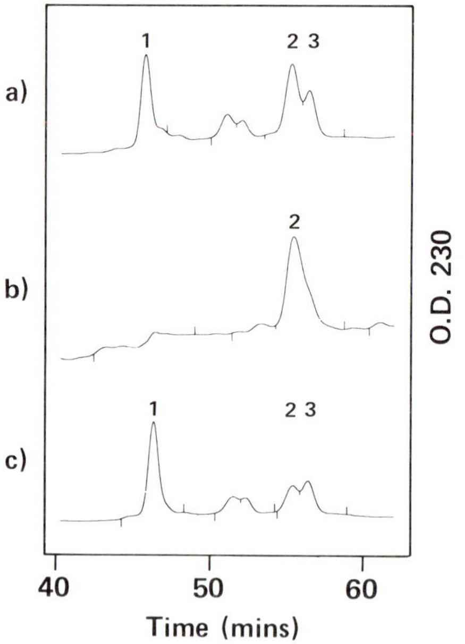

Fig. 5 Reverse-phase HPLC analysis of immunopurified recombinant IFN-α_2. (a) Profile of purified IFN-α_2. Peak 1 corresponds to oxidized IFN-α_2, peak 2 represents partially reduced IFN-α_2 and peak 3 a 14,500 M_r degradation product. (b) Sample reduced by 100 mM 2-mercaptoethanol. (c) Reduced sample reoxidized by dialysis against aerated phosphate buffered saline.

oxidized form of IFN-α_2 can be reduced by 2-mercaptoethanol to the partially-reduced form (Fig. 5b) and subsequently partially reoxidized by air oxidation (Fig. 5c). A 14500 M_r degradation product of IFN-α_2 is also resolved by our standard HPLC running conditions (peak 3, Fig. 5).

F Peptide Mapping

The state of the disulphide bonds in a protein can be determined by reverse-phase HPLC of tryptic or cyanogen bromide digests with or without prior reduction of disulphide bonds and was the technique used for the initial assignment of disulphides in IFN-α_2 (Wetzel, 1981). The technique is also useful to confirm programmed changes within analogue proteins where such changes are beyond the reach of *N*-terminal protein sequence identification.

G Spectral Analysis

A wide variety of spectroscopic techniques, such as fluorescence spectroscopy, circular dichroism and nuclear magnetic resonance, may be utilized for comparing structures of analogue proteins. X-ray crystallography provides the ultimate tool for the conformational analysis of analogues. However, the majority of techniques that provide detailed information require substantial quantities of homogeneous protein and considerable input of research time. Consequently, they may only be appropriate for analogue proteins being considered for commercial development.

H Summary

Immunoaffinity purification does not guarantee a monocomponent product and no single physico-chemical technique adequately characterizes a recombinant protein. PAGE-SDS and reverse-phase HPLC are probably the methods of choice for an initial assessment of product quality. The application of additional methods is desirable but must be considered in the light of limited resources, and a detailed characterization is probably only possible for analogues that show interesting biological properties and provide a lead for further analogue design.

VII BIOLOGICAL EVALUATION

The biological objectives of the structure–function programme were twofold. Firstly, to improve our very limited understanding of the mechanism of action of the interferons, and secondly to produce a modified interferon for therapeutic use that is superior to those presently available. Clearly the latter aim is extremely speculative and ambitious, and is complicated by the fact that it is not always clear which of the many *in vitro* effects of interferon are responsible for its *in vivo* activities. This is particularly apparent in the case of the antitumour response which is now well-documented for certain types of cancer. This dilemma poses a real problem for the clinician, who has to decide whether to use interferon as an antiproliferative or immunomodulatory agent.

With these problems in mind, we chose as a broad objective the separation of the major biological activities of interferon in the hope that this approach would produce therapeutically useful interferons with novel combinations of actions or with increased selectivity of action. At the outset of our programme there was no hard evidence that a separation of activities was possible, but it has since emerged that a species of human interferon-α, IFN-αJ, has potent antiviral and antiproliferative activity but is unable to stimulate natural killer cell activity (Ortaldo *et al.*, 1984). Thus, we can be confident that a dissociation of activities is an achievable target.

Initially, attention was concentrated on the three best-characterized biological effects of interferon

(1) Antiviral activity (WISH cells/EMC virus).
(2) Antiproliferative activity (Daudi cells).
(3) Stimulation of natural killer cell activity (Raji cells/human peripheral blood lymphocytes).

Many groups have developed sensitive assays to measure each of these activities, but the testing of interferon analogues did present some special problems. First of all, the assays had to be automated as far as possible so that large numbers of samples could be tested over a wide concentration range. In addition, it was important to determine the minimum level of purification of analogue that was compatible with the assays. The ability to assay crude lysates depends on a number of factors including the sensitivity of the assay, the expression level of the bacterial interferon and the effects of contaminating bacterial proteins. Toxic effects of bacterial contaminants were most apparent in the Daudi growth inhibition assay, but these were eradicated by a partial purification schedule of centrifugation, TCA precipitation and gel filtration, which gave a product that was at best 0.1–1% pure. Subsequently most analogues were also purified on monoclonal antibody affinity supports. In most instances the degree of purity of the sample did not significantly affect the ratios between titres in the human antiviral, antiproliferative and natural-killer-cell-stimulating bioassays (Fig. 6a). Therefore, the presence of bacterial contaminants did not preclude initial structure–activity interpretations.

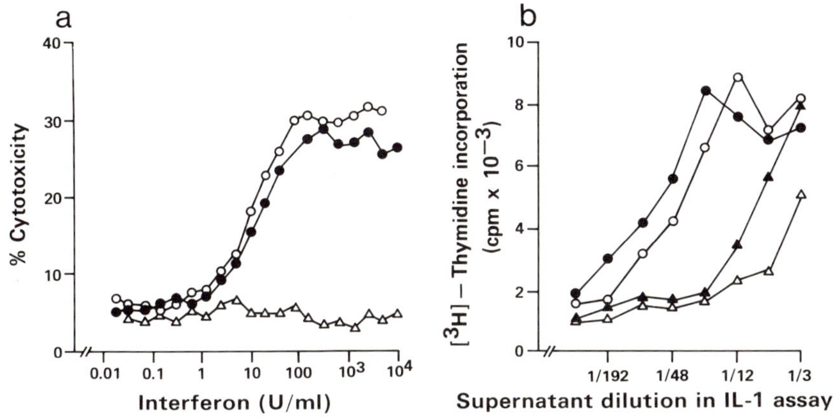

Fig. 6 (a) Stimulation of natural killer-cell activity by interferon. Human PBL were incubated with interferon overnight prior to a 4-hour ^{51}Cr-release cytotoxicity assay using Raji cells at an effector-to-target-cell ratio of 50:1. Monoclonal antibody purified IFN-α_2 (●), approximately 0.1% pure IFN-α_2 (○), 'blank' extract (△) processed in the same way as the crude IFN-α_2 and tested at equivalent protein concentration. (b) Effect of IFN-α_2 on LPS-induced IL-1 secretion. Incorporation of [^{3}H]thymidine by BALB/c thymocytes in the presence of phytohaemagglutinin and dilutions of monocyte culture supernatants. Monocytes were stimulated with 0.1 μg/ml LPS (△) after previous incubation with IFN-α_2 at 100 U/ml (▲), 1000 U/ml (●) or 10,000 U/ml (○).

During 1983 it became apparent that topical application of interferon for prophylaxis of respiratory viral infections caused inflammation of the nasal epithelium and submucosa (Hayden *et al.*, 1983). For the first time this gave a clear indication of what would constitute an improved interferon in the clinic and thus we decided to modify our testing procedure to try to find an interferon analogue with potent antiviral activity but which lacked this unacceptable side-effect. Interleukin-1 (IL-1) appears to play a major role in the inflammatory response (Marx, 1983). It stimulates fibroblasts to proliferate (Schmidt *et al.*, 1981) and to produce collagenase and plasminogen activator (Hamilton *et al.*, 1982), possibly contributing to tissue remodelling and fibrosis. It also stimulates synovial cells to release collagenase and prostaglandins (Mizel *et al.*, 1981).

Therefore, it is possible that the local inflammatory effect of interferons in the upper respiratory tract might be mediated by IL-1. Further weight was added to this hypothesis by the report that interferon enhances production of IL-1 from human monocytes (Arenzana-Seisdedos and Virelizier, 1983; Boraschi *et al.*, 1984). It has been suggested that the pyrexia associated with interferon therapy may be mediated through endogenous pyrogen (Scott *et al.*, 1983), which is thought to be identical to IL-1. There are a number of similarities between the effects in humans of interferon-α and endogenous pyrogen/IL-1: (i) both are pyrogenic; (ii) both cause falls in plasma zinc levels (Scott *et al.*, 1983); and (iii) both cause increases in the acute phase protein, serum amyloid A (Maury *et al.*, 1983). Thus, there may be a link between interferon-α and IL-1 in relation to the pyrexia and local inflammation observed in the clinic.

An *in vitro* bioassay was established in which human monocytes isolated from peripheral blood were incubated with interferon analogues for 24 hours. After this pre-incubation stage, monocyte cultures were stimulated by a low dose of lipopolysaccharide for a further 24 hours. Supernatants were then removed and tested for IL-1 activity in a thymocyte proliferation assay. All the interferon samples tested were purified on monoclonal antibody affinity supports. Typical dose–response curves obtained with IFN-α_2 are shown in Fig. 6b.

VIII STRUCTURE–ACTIVITY RESULTS

IFN-α_2 is a single polypeptide chain of 165 amino acid residues (Streuli *et al.*, 1980) cross-linked by two disulphide bridges (Wetzel, 1981) (Fig. 7). When

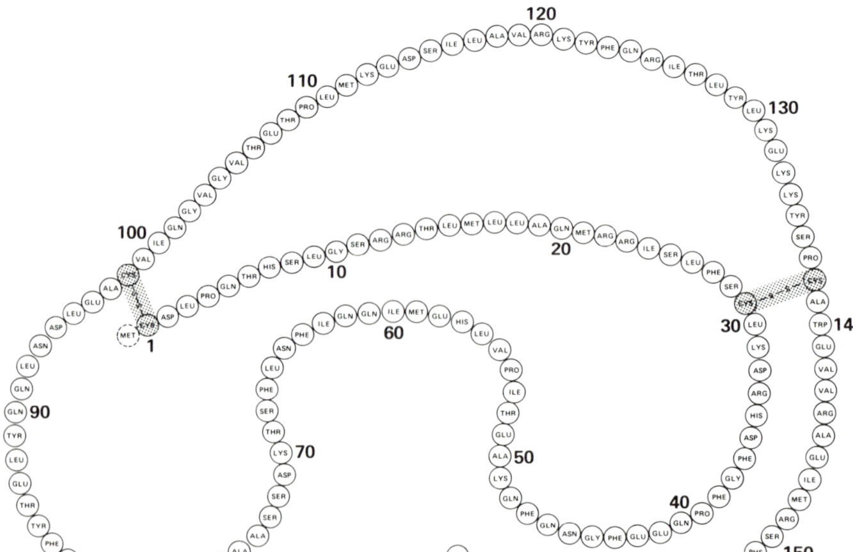

Fig. 7 Amino acid sequence of IFN-α_2 indicating disulphide bridges.

we set out, IFN-α_2 was already known to be one of a family of structurally closely homologous human IFN-α proteins (Goeddel *et al.*, 1981; Weissmann *et al.*, 1982; Allen and Fantes, 1980) and to bear significant homology to the single known species of human IFN-β (Taniguchi *et al.*, 1980). Several theoretical models of secondary (Hayes, 1980; Wetzel *et al.*, 1982; DeGrado *et al.*, 1982) and tertiary (Sternberg and Cohen, 1982; Zav'yalov and Denesyuk, 1982) conformations existed, but no reliable 3-dimensional structure based on X-ray crystallographic data was available. In consequence, most of our ideas derived from considerations of the sequence of IFN-α_2 and from the differences and similarities in sequence between the various human IFN species. Some of the results described below have been summarized elsewhere (Camble *et al.*, 1985).

A Amino- and Carboxyl-Terminal Regions

1 C-terminal truncated analogues

Several reports already indicated that the 13 amino acid residues at the carboxy-terminus of IFN-α_2 were not essential for biological activity. Limited thermolysin digestion of purified IFN-αA had yielded IFN-αA(1–152) (with an additional peptide bond cleaved at position 109) which retained almost all the antiviral activity of the intact protein (Wetzel *et al.*, 1982), and two purified active natural leukocyte IFN proteins had been shown to lack the 10 carboxy-terminal residues (Evinger *et al.*, 1981; Levy *et al.*, 1981). Expression in *E. coli* of genes for truncated IFN-αA(1–154) (Franke *et al.*, 1982) and for a hybrid of IFN-αA(1–154) followed by nine unrelated residues encoded by the β-lactamase gene of pBR322 (Chang *et al.*, 1983) had also given biologically active products, but in each case increased susceptibility to proteolytic degradation in the bacterial host was suspected.

As an early test of the ability of interferon proteins to survive our planned routine for expression, extraction and size-exclusion chromatography, we constructed plasmids expressing genes for IFN-α_2(1–160), IFN-α_2(1–155) and IFN-α_2(1-147). The first two each provided a single major new protein band on PAGE-SDS of extracts from radio-labelled minicells; *E. coli* lysate supernatants showed antiviral and NK2-IRMA titres within a factor of 3–4 of those shown by IFN-α_2. No activity or new radio-labelled protein could be detected in extracts of cells containing the gene for IFN-α_2(1–147). These results seemed consistent with the literature and supported the viability of our overall approach to analogue production. IFN-α_2(1–160) and IFN-α_2(1–155) showed no significant differences from IFN-α_2 itself in the ratios between antiviral, antiproliferative, NK-cell-stimulating and NK2-IRMA titres, either with gel-filtered samples, or later with NK2-Sepharose purified samples.

2 N-terminal truncated analogues

To our knowledge, no information existed in 1982 on the importance of the *N*-terminal residues of IFN-α_2 for activity, apart from a comment in a patent application (Weissmann, 1981) that the first nine residues of IFN-α_1 are not necessary for antiviral activity. We found that extracts containing the target analogue IFN-α_2(4–165) showed activity similar to IFN-α_2 in all three bioassays and cross-reacted with NK2, indicating that the first three residues of IFN-α_2 and the integrity of the Cysl-Cys98 disulphide bridge are not critical for activity. Other workers have drawn similar conclusions from chemical modification studies with purified IFN-αA (Wetzel *et al.*, 1982; Morehead *et al.*, 1984), from complete chemical synthesis of biologically active [Ser^1]IFN-α_1 (Merrifield, 1983), and from construction of recombinants expressing IFN-α_1(5–166) and IFN-α_2(5–62)/α_1(64–166) (Lydon *et al.*, 1985).

Genes encoding IFN-α_2(10–165) and IFN-α_2(12–165) produced very low levels of protein product as a result, we believe, of a block to gene transcription or translation arising from undesirable secondary structure formation in the gene or mRNA. Extracts of both analogues did give just-detectable levels of antiviral activity, but redesigned DNA constructs expressing at higher levels are required before firm conclusions can be drawn.

Genes for IFN-α_2(14–165), IFN-α_2(16–165) and IFN-α_2(21–165) gave good levels of protein product. All three truncated products were antiviral inactive but still cross-reacted with NK2 monoclonal antibody. The absence of biological activity in target analogues IFN-α_2(14–165) and IFN-α_2(16–165) seemed to contradict predictions that the latter ought to be active (Arnheiter *et al.*, 1983; Zoon and Wetzel, 1984). However, NK2-purified samples of all three truncated analogues showed a single major product with identical mobility on PAGE-SDS, a mobility corresponding to that of an impurity (MW about 14,500) observed in varying amounts in some batches of IFN-α_2. Together with other evidence, this suggested that the different truncated analogues may each be degraded rapidly to a common, shorter product, and we should conclude nothing for the time being about the biological activity of IFN-α_2(16–165). Clearly, *N*-terminal sequence analysis is indicated as the next step in characterization of these analogues.

We can say, however, that our results do not support the suggestion (Lydon *et al.*, 1985) that the first 15 residues from the amino terminus may contribute to the epitope recognized by the NK2 monoclonal antibody. The NK2-purified products from IFN-α_2(14–165), IFN-α_2(16–165) and IFN-α_2(21–165) gave specific activities of 4×10^8, 2×10^8 and 4×10^8 NK2-IRMA units/mg of protein respectively. Indeed, NK2 still recognized and was used to purify the badly degraded heterogeneous protein product obtained from a gene for IFN-α_2 (29–165).

3 N-*and* C-*terminal truncated analogues*

Combining the individual truncations compatible with retention of biological activity, genes for IFN-α_2(4–160) and IFN-α_2(4–155) produced reasonable titres of biologically and immunologically active proteins. IFN-α_2(4–160) showed no significant separation of antiviral from antiproliferative or NK-cell-stimulating activities relative to IFN-α_2. However, IFN-α_2(4–155) (specific activity 2×10^8 antiviral IU/mg of protein, 6×10^8 NK2-IRMA U/mg) showed a consistent 10-fold increase over IFN-α_2 in the number of antiviral units required to produce a 50% inhibition of Daudi cell proliferation. This apparent decrease in relative antiproliferative potency was obtained with samples prepared by size-exclusion chromatography and with samples purified on NK2-Sepharose, starting from lysate supernatants or guanidine hydrochloride extracts of cell pastes from two different strains of *E. coli*. This significant but by no means dramatic separation of different activities is the largest we have found among all the different analogues we have examined. In general, for all other analogues described in this review, it can be assumed that the level of antiviral activity reflects activity in the other bioprofiling assays.

4 N-*terminal substitutions*

To avoid the complications of gene non-expression or protein degradation associated with truncated analogues, substitution with completely unrelated sequences was used to probe the importance of *N*-terminal region amino acids for biological activity. Replacement of residues 2–7 (Asp-Leu-Pro-Gln-Thr-His) of IFN-α_2 with residues 2–7 (Tyr-Cys-Gln-Asp-Pro-Tyr) from human IFN-γ (Gray and Goeddel, 1982) gave [Tyr^2, Cys^3, Gln^4, Asp^5, Pro^6, Tyr^7]IFN-α_2 or [$\gamma(2–7)^{2-7}$]IFN-α_2. This analogue showed activities (1.3×10^8 antiviral IU/mg of protein, 9×10^8 NK2-IRMA U/mg), similar to IFN-α_2 (see Table I).

Substitution of amino acids 10–15 of IFN-α_2 by alanine residues to give [Ala^{10-15}]IFN-α_2 reduced biological potency (specific activity 1×10^6 antiviral IU/mg), but produced only a modest drop in NK2-cross-reactivity (5×10^8 NK2-IRMA U/mg). This 100-fold reduction in biological activity still represents a potency on human cells only slightly below that of IFN-α_1 (see Table I). Thus none of the specific amino acid side-chains in residues 2–7 or 10–15 of IFN-α_2 can be critical for activity.

5 N-*terminal IFN-α_2/α_1 hybrids*

Using analogues expressed from hybrid cDNA genes, the low specific antiviral activity on human cells of IFN-α_1 relative to IFN-α_2 has been attributed to the 12 amino acid differences in the sequences of the first 62 residues from the *N*-terminus (Fig. 8) (Streuli *et al.*, 1981). In an attempt to define further which of these 12 residues is responsible for the drop in potency, we prepared several new IFN-α_2/α_1 hybrids using synthetic genes. [Glu^5, Asp^{10}, Ser^{11}]IFN-α_2 or [α_1(1–11)$^{1-11}$]IFN-α_2, incorporating the three amino acid differences in the first 21 residues, was biologically and immunologically similar to IFN-α_2

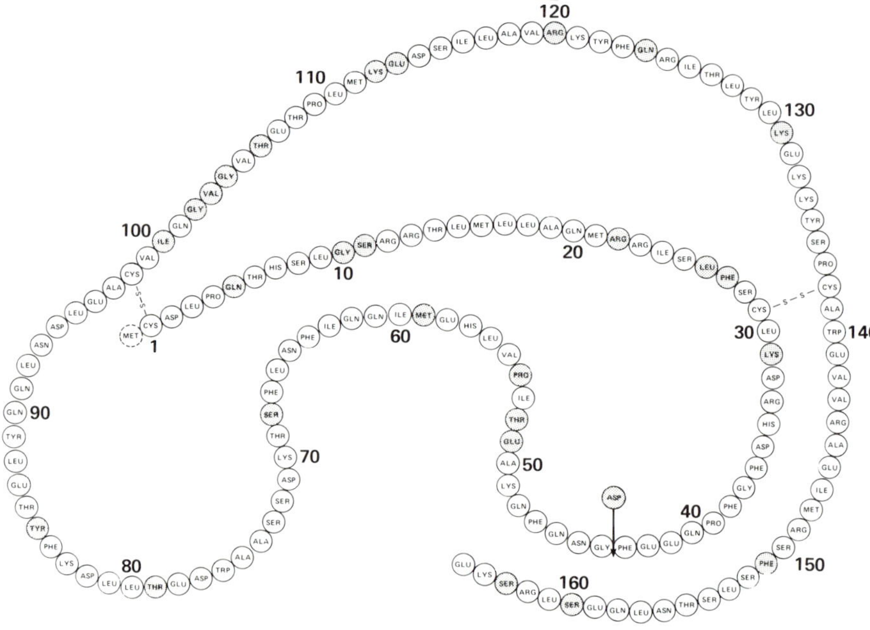

Fig. 8 Sequence of IFN-α_2 indicating residues changed in IFN-α_1.

(4 × 10^8 antiviral IU/mg, 6 × 10^9 NK2-IRMA U/mg). The expected residue changes in this analogue were confirmed by gas-phase *N*-terminal amino acid sequencing (Hunkapiller and Hood, 1983; performed for us by Dr H. Gregory of this Department). Almost identical activity profiles were shown by endo-Asp^{43a}IFN-α_2 and endo-Asp^{43a} [α_1(1–11)$^{1-11}$]IFN-α_2, which contain the additional aspartic acid residue inserted at position 44 in IFN-α_1 and all other human IFN-α species except IFN-α_2.

The only difference between IFN-α_2 and IFN-α_1 from residues 56–62 is a methionine to leucine change at position 59 (IFN-α_2 numbering). [Leu^{59}]IFN-α_2 (2 × 10^8 antiviral IU/mg; 1 × 10^9 NK2-IRMA U/mg) again proved to be very like IFN-α_2. Therefore, the low antiviral potency of IFN-α_1 results either from one or more of the remaining seven residue changes between positions 22 and 55, or from some combination of these residues with the five we had already examined.

As a final probe we recently prepared [Glu^5, Ser^{27}, Met^{31}, Leu^{59}]IFN-α_2, an analogue containing four residues from IFN-α_1 that do not occur in those positions in any other species of human IFN-α; in addition, those positions are conserved in other human IFN-α species. This analogue showed NK2-activity similar to IFN-α_2(1.2 $\times$ 10^9 NK2-IRMA U/mg), but first results indicated an antiviral potency closer to that of IFN-α_1 (specific antiviral activity 5–10 $\times$ 10^6 IU/mg). This suggests that if a single residue is indeed responsible for the relatively low specific activity of IFN-α_1 on human cells, then Ser27 or Met31 could be prime candidates. In particular, Met31 is surrounded by four strictly conserved residues (see section VIII (E)), and

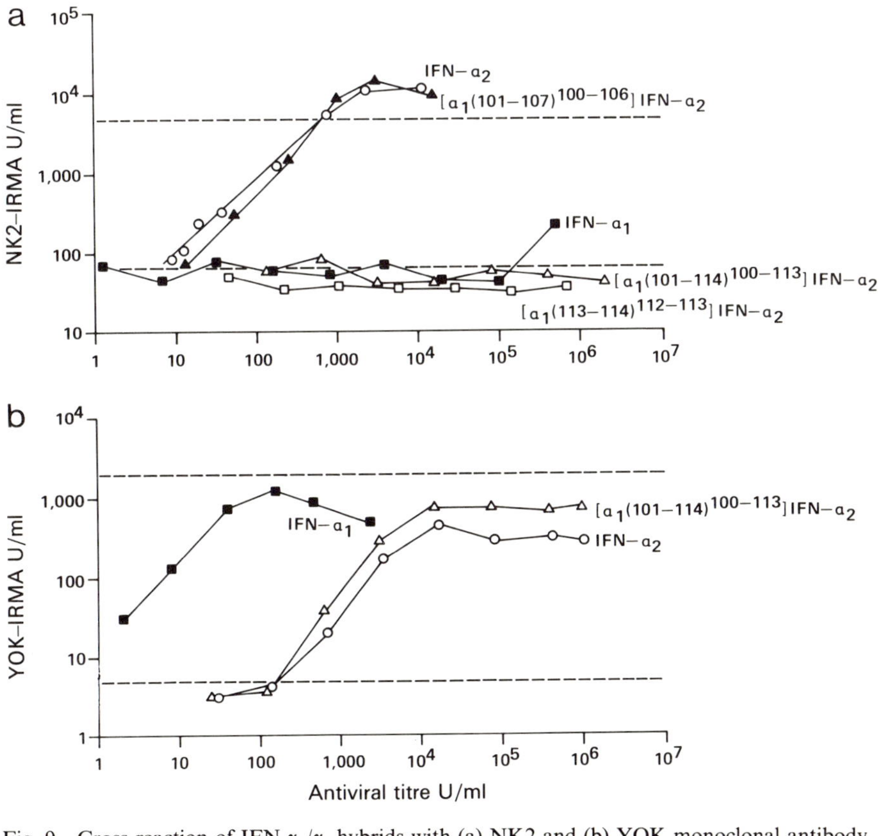

Fig. 9 Cross-reaction of IFN-α_2/α_1 hybrids with (a) NK2 and (b) YOK monoclonal antibody.

TABLE I Specific Activities of Purified IFNs and Hybrid Analogues

	Specific activity (U/mg)		
Target Protein	Antiviral	NK_2–IRMA	YOK–IRMA
IFN-α_2	2×10^8	2.5×10^9	7×10^6
IFN-α_1	8×10^6	4×10^3	1.5×10^8
[$\alpha_1(101–114)^{100–113}$]IFN-$\alpha_2$	6×10^8	$< 1.4 \times 10^{4a}$	2×10^7
[$\alpha_1(101–107)^{100–106}$]IFN-$\alpha_2$	2×10^8	1×10^9	8×10^6
[$\alpha_1(113–114)^{112–113}$]IFN-$\alpha_2$	2×10^8	$< 1.3 \times 10^{4a}$	1×10^7
[$\gamma(98–114)^{98–114}$]IFN-α_2	2×10^8	$< 4.3 \times 10^{4a}$	8×10^6
[$\gamma(98–107)^{98–107}$]IFN-α_2	1×10^8	1×10^9	7×10^6
[$\gamma(95–101)^{101–107}$]IFN-α_2	5×10^8	2×10^9	1×10^7

[a] No activity detected at the highest concentrations used.

lysine is found at this position not only in all other human IFN-α species but also in human IFN-β.

B The Region of Residues 98–114

1 IFN-α_2/α_1 hybrids and the epitope for NK2 monoclonal antibody

As described above (Section V (E)), in early work we found that, whereas IFN-α_2 was recognized by the commercially available NK2 monoclonal antibody, IFN-α_1 was barely detectable in the NK2-IRMA at 10^4 times higher antiviral concentrations (Fig. 9a). Given the low specific antiviral activity of IFN-α_1 on human cells (Table I), this corresponds to at least 10^5 times higher protein concentration. Not surprisingly, IFN-α_1 is not retained and cannot be purified on NK2-Sepharose. IFN-α_1 differs from IFN-α_2 at 27 positions and also has an additional aspartic acid residue inserted at position 44 (Fig. 8). From the results presented in the last section (VIII (A5)), it seems clear that at least 7 of the 12 changes in the *N*-terminal 62 residues are not involved in this dramatic loss of cross-reactivity. The observations with truncated analogues (Section VIII (A1)) suggest that the two changes towards the *C*-terminus are also not important.

Seven of the remaining 18 differences are concentrated between positions 100 and 113 of IFN-α_2. The hybrid analogue [Met^{100}, Glu^{102}, Glu^{103}, Arg^{104}, Gly^{106}, Asn^{112}, Ala^{113}]IFN-α_2, or [$\alpha_1(101–114)^{100–113}$]IFN-$\alpha_2$, was prepared and showed biological activity indistinguishable from IFN-α_2, as would be predicted from published data (Streuli *et al.*, 1981), but was not recognized by NK2 (Fig. 9a, Table I). The residues critical for antibody recognition were defined further with two more hybrid analogues. [$\alpha_1(101–107)^{100–106}$]IFN-$\alpha_2$

behaved like IFN-α_2 in every respect, but [Asn^{112}, Ala^{113}]IFN-2α containing just two changes was again not recognized by the antibody (Fig. 9a, Table I). We conclude that the presence of this Asn-Ala sequence in IFN-α_1 is sufficient to account for its lack of reaction with NK2 and that some part of the corresponding Lys-Glu dipeptide in IFN-α_2 probably makes an important contribution to the epitope for this monoclonal antibody.

The synthetic hexapeptide derivative Acetyl-Leu-Met-Lys-Glu-Asp-Ser-NH_2, corresponding to residues 110–115 of IFN-α_2, failed even at high concentrations to displace IFN-α_2 from NK2-Sepharose or to compete with IFN-α_2 in the NK2-IRMA. This suggests that the Lys-Glu sequence does not represent the complete epitope for NK2.

Two recent observations by other workers are relevant to these results. First, a critical part of the epitope for another, independently generated, monoclonal antibody LI-1 has also been localized to the Glu113 residue of IFN-αA (Trown *et al.*, 1985). Second, studies with CNBr cleavage fragments of IFN-α_2 suggest that part of the epitope for NK2 may reside in the polypeptide comprising the amino-terminal 15 amino acids linked to residues 60–110 by a disulphide bridge (Lydon *et al.*, 1985).

IFN-α_1 is recognized by the more recently available YOK monoclonal antibody (Fig. 9b, Table I). IFN-α_2 binds less well to this antibody but can still be purified on YOK-Sepharose. With this antibody, the hybrid analogue [α_1(101–114)$^{100-113}$]IFN-α_2 behaves like IFN-α_2 rather than IFN-α_1. Indeed, most analogues examined seem to be recognized by this antibody in a similar fashion to IFN-α_2; a few are unreactive but none demonstrated the increased affinity shown by IFN-α_1. For this reason YOK-Sepharose was very useful for purification of those analogues that did not cross-react with NK2.

2 *IFN-α_2/γ hybrids*

Substitution of completely unrelated sequences from IFN-γ (Gray and Goeddel, 1982) into positions 98–114 of IFN-α_2 (Fig. 10) had little effect on biological activity (Table I), indicating that none of the specific amino acid side-chains in this region are important for activity. In [γ(98–114)$^{98-114}$]IFN-α_2 and [γ(98–107)$^{98-107}$]IFN-α_2 the Cys98 residue of IFN-α_2 is substituted. Activity in these analogues reinforced the earlier conclusion from *N*-terminal truncated analogues that the integrity of the 1–98 disulphide bridge is not important for activity. The pattern of cross-reactivity of these analogues with NK2 (Table I) is consistent with the conclusion drawn from IFN-α_2/α_1 hybrids about the importance of residues 112–113 for antibody recognition.

All the data in Fig. 9 and Table I were compiled with immunoaffinity-purified samples whose behaviour on PAGE-SDS is illustrated in Fig. 11. Under reducing conditions all analogues gave one major protein band.

Target Analogue	Position																
	98	99	100	101	102	103	104	105	106	107	108	109	110	111	112	113	114
IFN – α_2	Cys	Val	Ile	Gln	Gly	Val	Gly	Val	Thr	Glu	Thr	Pro	Leu	Met	Lys	Glu	Asp
$[\gamma(98-114)^{98-114}]$	Leu	Thr	Asn	Tyr	Ser	Val	Thr	Asp	Leu	Asn	Val	Gln	Arg	Lys	Ala	Ile	His
$[\gamma(98-107)^{98-107}]$	Leu	Thr	Asn	Tyr	Ser	Val	Thr	Asp	Leu	Asn							
$[\gamma(95-101)^{101-107}]$				Phe	Glu	Lys	Leu	Thr	Asn	Tyr							

Fig. 10 IFN-γ sequences substituted between positions 98–114 of IFN-α_2.

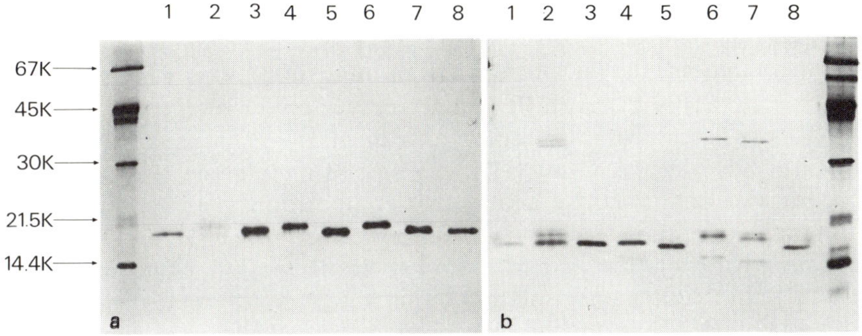

Fig. 11 PAGE-SDS electrophoresis of IFN-α_2, IFN-α_1 and analogues after immunoaffinity purification on NK2- or YOK-Sepharose (a) In the presence and (b) in the absence of 2 mercaptoethanol. Lanes: **1**, IFN-α_2; **2**, IFN-α_1; **3**, $[\alpha_1(101\text{–}114)^{100\text{–}113}]$IFN-$\alpha_2$; **4**, $[\alpha_1(101\text{–}107)^{100\text{–}106}]$ IFN-α_2; **5**, $[\alpha_1(113\text{–}114)^{112\text{–}113}]$IFN-$\alpha_2$; **6**, $[\gamma(98\text{–}114)^{98\text{–}114}]$IFN-$\alpha_2$; **7**, $[\gamma(98\text{–}107)^{98\text{–}107}]$IFN-$\alpha_2$; **8**, $[\gamma(95\text{–}101)^{101\text{–}107}]$IFN-$\alpha_2$. Target protein sequences in lanes 2, 6 and 7 contain 5, 3 and 3 cysteine residues respectively. The slower running "spots" in (b) at the outer edges of lanes 1 and 8 probably arise from reducing agent present in marker protein lanes diffusing across to the nearside of the analogue lanes and partially reducing disulphide bridges.

However, under non-reducing conditions multiple monomer bands (incomplete or incorrect disulphide bridge formation?) and probable oligomer species can be detected. Interestingly, oligomer bands are most prominent in those analogues that contain an odd number of cysteine residues.

3 *Deletion of residues*

As a final demonstration of the unimportance of this region for activity, the analogue des(101–110)IFN-α_2, in which the decapeptide sequence of IFN-α_2 from positions 101–110 has been deleted and Ile100 is linked directly to Met111, was prepared and showed all four biological activities and reacted with NK2. This remarkable result suggests that the whole region might form a loop rather as illustrated in one available conformational model (Sternberg and Cohen, 1982).

C Specific Types of Amino Acid Residues

Glycine residues often play an important role in the 3-dimensional conformation adopted by proteins and peptides by promoting the formation of turns in the polypeptide chain. When alanine residues were substituted for all five glycine residues in IFN-α_2, introducing both chirality and significant conformational restraint at these positions, the activities of $[\text{Ala}^{10,37,44,102,104}]$IFN-$\alpha_2$ were indistinguishable from IFN-α_2 (specific activity 2.8×10^8 antiviral IU/mg; 1.5×10^9 NK2-IRMA U/mg). This is consistent with the fact that none of the five glycine residues in IFN-α_2 is conserved in all other human IFN-α species.

Replacement of all five methionine residues in IFN-α_2 with leucine in [$Leu^{16,21,59,111,148}$]IFN-α_2 gave a 10-fold decrease in both biological activity and in NK2-cross-reactivity (specific activity 1.1×10^7 antiviral IU/mg, 1.5×10^8 NK2-IRMA U/mg). The absence of methionine residues in this analogue was confirmed by amino acid composition analysis. Single substitutions of methionine by leucine at positions 16, 21, 59 and 111 gave analogues with specific activities similar to IFN-α_2 (a clone expressing [Leu^{148}]IFN-α_2 was never isolated). This retention of biological activity in an analogue lacking methionine residues provided a first step towards possible protein semi-synthetic manipulation of the IFN-α_2 molecule (see Section IX).

Though not conserved among human IFN-α species, the three lysine residues in positions 31, 131 and 133 of IFN-α_2 might form a basic cluster in one conformational model (Sternberg and Cohen, 1982). When arginine residues were substituted at all three positions, [$Arg^{31,131,133}$]IFN-α_2 showed good activity (about 3×10^7 antiviral IU/mg, 7×10^8 NK2-IRMA U/mg).

D The 29–138 Disulphide Bridge

Interest in this disulphide bridge first arose from a consideration of homologies between sequences of Type I interferons. The four cysteine residues in IFN-α_2 are conserved among all known species of human IFN-α; human IFN-β contains only three cysteines, but two of these are found in positions homologous to Cys29 and Cys138 in IFN-α_2. As these two cysteines form a disulphide bridge in IFN-αA (Wetzel, 1981) it seemed likely that this disulphide bridge could be conserved among human IFN-α and IFN-β species. The known sensitivity to reducing agents of antiviral activity in IFN-α and IFN-β might then be explained if the integrity of this conserved disulphide bridge was critical for biological activity.

The first evidence to support this picture came with the isolation of a mutant recombinant IFN-β in which one of the two conserved cysteines was replaced by a tyrosine residue and which was devoid of antiviral activity (Shepard *et al.*, 1981). Clear demonstration that this disulphide bridge is indeed essential for antiviral activity and for stabilizing the active conformation of IFN-αA seemed to be provided by elegant chemical modification experiments (Wetzel *et al.*, 1982; 1983; Morehead *et al.*, 1984). However, it has also been reported that proteolytic digestion of IFN-α_2 can yield a biologically active fragment consisting only of residues 1–110 (Ackerman *et al.*, 1984) that cannot contain the 29–138 disulphide cross-link.

134 135 136 137 138 139 140 141 142
—Lys—Tyr —Ser —Pro—Cys—Ala —Trp—Glu —Val—
|
—Ser —Leu —Phe—Ser —Cys—Leu—Lys—Asp—Arg—
25 26 27 28 29 30 31 32 33

Fig. 12 Amino acid sequences around the Cys29–Cys138 disulphide bridge.

We looked first at the importance of the precise position of these two cysteine residues (Fig. 12). Four analogues were designed in which each cysteine was moved one position along the sequence in either direction. [Cys^{28}, Ser^{29}]IFN-α_2, [Leu^{29}, Cys^{30}]IFN-α_2 and [Ala^{138}, Cys^{139}]IFN-α_2 were each devoid of biological activity on human cells, but all three gave typical titres in the NK2-IRMA. The NK2-activity of [Ala^{138}, Cys^{139}]IFN-α_2 was also relatively labile and titre was greatly reduced during processing to give profiling samples. The fourth target analogue, [Cys^{137}, Pro^{138}]IFN-α_2, failed to accumulate any new protein in minicells. This suggests that the stability of the protein products in *E. coli* is more sensitive to changes around Cys138 than around Cys29. Displacement of the Cys29 by two positions along the chain with [Cys^{27}, Phe^{28}, Ser^{29}]IFN-α_2 and [Leu^{29}, Lys^{30}, Cys^{31}]IFN-α_2 also gave biologically inactive NK2-positive products.

Interpretation of these results depends on the state of the cysteine residues. At one extreme the protein chain may fold as in IFN-α_2; in this case, most nearby amino acids need not change their juxtapositions relative to each other, but a disulphide bridge would not form between the displaced cysteine residues (illustrated very schematically in Fig. 13a for [Cys^{27}, Ser^{28}]IFN-α_2 and not intended to imply that the two segments of polypeptide chain are really orientated parallel to each other). Alternatively, a disulphide bridge may form between the two cysteines; in this case at least some nearby amino acids must change their relative juxtapositions (Fig. 13b). The problem was complicated further by the emerging evidence from our own and published data (Pestka *et al.*, 1983) of a lack of complete fidelity in disulphide bond formation in immunoaffinity-purified recombinant IFN-α_2 itself. What is clear is that none of these cysteine movements makes a great difference to recognition by the NK2 monoclonal antibody.

[Cys^{28}, Ser^{29}]IFN-α_2 in particular involves a very conservative change in primary structure, in which a thiol and a hydroxyl group have been exchanged between two adjacent residues. That such a minor change leads to complete loss of all biological activity indicated just how critical the disulphide, or the conformation of residues in the proximity of the disulphide, must be for activity. The non-essential nature of the neighbouring Ser28 and

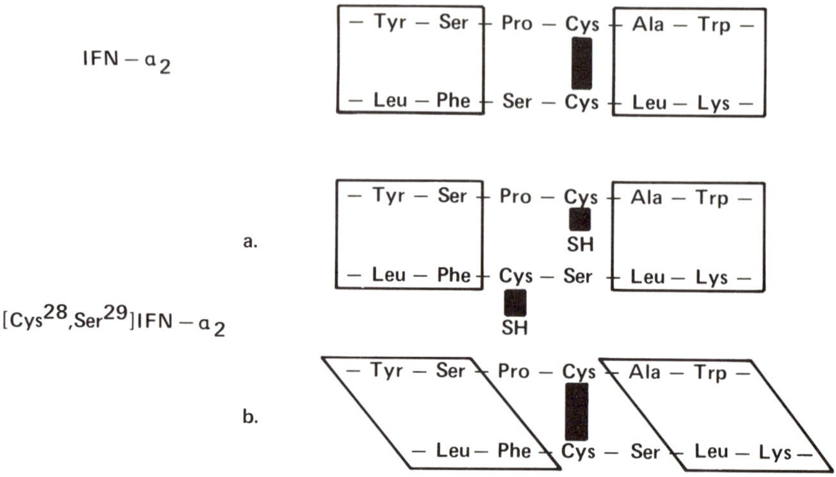

Fig. 13 Schematic representation of possible effects of cysteine residue displacement on juxtapositions of neighbouring residues.

Pro137 residues, as distinct from the cysteine residues, was shown with $[Ala^{28}]IFN\text{-}\alpha_2$ and $[Ala^{137}]IFN\text{-}\alpha_2$, both of which showed typical activities (about 1×10^8 antiviral IU/mg, 1.3×10^9 NK2-IRMA U/mg and 1×10^8 antiviral IU/mg, 1.1×10^9 NK2-IRMA U/mg respectively). The Ala30 residue is considered in Section VIII (E).

In an attempt to distinguish between the two possibilities in Fig. 13a and b, we prepared $[Ser^{29,138}]IFN\text{-}\alpha_2$, in which both cysteine residues are substituted by serine and there is no possibility of forming a disulphide bridge. Somewhat to our surprise, this analogue showed consistent substantial activity in all four biological assays (about 8×10^6 antiviral IU/mg, 2.5×10^8 NK2-IRMA U/mg). This represents some 4% of the specific antiviral activity of IFN-α_2, but is still comparable with the specific activity of IFN-α_1 on human cells. The sequence of the cloned synthetic gene for this analogue has been confirmed, and comparison of the amino acid ratios in acid hydrolysates of performic-acid-oxidized samples of purified $[Ser^{29,138}]IFN\text{-}\alpha_2$ and IFN-α_2 show the required increase in serine and decrease in cysteic acid content in the analogue.* The results with this analogue indicate clearly that the integrity of the 29–138 disulphide crosslink in IFN-α_2 cannot be essential either for activity or for ensuring a biologically active conformation.

* These analyses were kindly performed for us by Moyra Simpson, Millipore, Waters Chromatography Division, Herriot-Watt University, Edinburgh, Scotland, on about 60 picomoles of protein using the new sensitive PICO-TAG method of amino acid analysis.

The decrease in potency in [$Ser^{29,138}$]IFN-α_2 may result from some slight distortion of surrounding conformation when two hydroxyl groups have to be accommodated in the space normally occupied by a disulphide bond. Reduced, *S*-alkylated derivatives of IFN-α_2, which would be even more sterically hindered, have been shown to be inactive (Morehead *et al.*, 1984). An alternative model might be that the IFN-α_2 protein chain has a spectrum of conformations open to it but that only those compatible jwith formation of the disulphide bridge produce biological activity. With IFN-α_2, when the disulphide bridge forms in *E. coli* or during isolation, the protein is effectively "trapped" into a limited sub-set of more biologically productive conformations and so shows high specific activity. In [$Ser^{29,138}$]IFN-α_2, the whole conformational spectrum would always remain available to the protein, so that it only has a fraction of the activity of IFN-α_2 corresponding to the fraction of time it spends in the disulphide-like conformation. In [Cys^{28}, Ser^{29}]IFN-α_2 and the other inactive cysteine-shifted analogues, formation of a disulphide bond might provide a 'conformational trap' limiting the analogues to a sub-set of biologically unproductive conformations. The unusual behaviour of purified IFN-α_2 during chemical reduction and re-oxidation under native and denaturing conditions (Morehead *et al.*, 1984) emphasizes the difficulty in interpreting structure–activity results involving this disulphide bridge.

We next prepared [Ser^{29}]IFN-α_2 and [Ser^{138}]IFN-α_2, in which just one of the two cysteines is replaced by a serine residue. Both analogues showed only a trace of antiviral activity (about 10^5 IU/mg maximum) but good NK2 reactivity (3×10^9 and 6×10^8 NK2-IRMA U/mg respectively). These results do not support the conformational trap model, since these analogues, like [$Ser^{29,138}$]IFN-α_2, cannot form an intramolecular disulphide bridge (unless it be with Cys1 or Cys98). The results could be consistent with the steric hindrance model, as a cysteine thiol group is more bulky than a second serine hydroxyl group. However, [Gly^{29}]IFN-α_2, which should be no more hindered than [$Ser^{29,138}$]IFN-α_2, also proved to be essentially antiviral inactive. Finally, we prepared [$Gly^{29,138}$]IFN-α_2, which was again biologically almost inactive (very approximately 5×10^3 antiviral IU/mg; 4×10^8 NK2-IRMA U/mg). During the writing of this review, a report appeared on the preparation by site-directed mutagenesis of the equivalent of [Ser^{29}]IFN-α_2 in a fusion protein of IFN-α_1 with nine additional amino acids at the *N*-terminus. This retained some 6% of the antiviral activity of the parent protein (Nisbet *et al.*, 1985).

We conclude that even though [$Ser^{28,138}$]IFN-α_2 demonstrates that biological activity can be retained in the absence of the Cys29–Cys138 disulphide bridge, this is a very special case and it is unlikely that high biological activity will be achieved in the absence of the stabilizing cross-link.

E Amino Acids Conserved Among Human Type I IFNs

Human IFN-α and IFN-β share similar biological profiles and appear to compete for the same target cell surface receptors (Branca and Baglioni, 1981; Aguet and Blanchard, 1981; Joshi *et al.*, 1982; Yonehara *et al.*, 1983; Merlin *et al.*, 1985). If a limited number of structural elements critical for biological activity do exist in IFN-α_2, then preferred places to look for them would be among the amino acid side-chains conserved or only conservatively substituted between all the human Type I IFN species.

Human IFN-α_2 and IFN-α_1 have the same amino acid residues in 138 positions. Across all human IFN-α sequences reported from either gene translation (see Weissmann *et al.*, 1982 for a review) or direct protein sequencing data (Allen and Fantes, 1980), there are still nearly 90 conserved residues. However, when the human IFN-β (Taniguchi *et al.*, 1980) is included the number of strictly conserved residues falls to just 35 (Fig. 14). It seemed unlikely that the size of this ultimately conserved group would fall much farther; the original comparison of IFN-α_1 and IFN-β (Taniguchi *et al.*, 1980) had revealed 49 conserved residues and the total had already fallen to 36 with the first publication of eight IFN-α sequences (Goeddel *et al.*, 1981). Changes at some other positions are highly conservative or only occur in just one IFN-α species, but we decided to focus first on this group of 35 strictly conserved residues. (Similar analyses have been recorded by Derynck *et al.*, (1982) and Content and Derynck (1983), but only sequence data from gene translation were considered.)

There was no reason to expect that all 35 conserved residues need be essential for function or for maintaining the active conformation of IFN-α_2. Indeed, conserved residues 3 and 161 could already be excluded by our observations of biological activity with *N*- and *C*-terminal truncated analogues. We planned to explore the remaining 31 amino acid positions (the two conserved cysteine residues in positions 29 and 138 were considered separately, see Section VIII (D) by preparing six analogues with clusters of 4 to 7 residues changed at a time. After this first scan, with luck, only the conserved residues in those analogues showing a loss or separation of activity need be studied individually or in combinations of smaller clusters. This strategy limited the number of analogues required in an initial survey and exploited the ease with which multiple changes could be attempted using the synthetic gene approach. In addition, it would reveal limitations in gene synthesis and cloning, product stability and structure–activity interpretation and so provide guidelines for future judgements on the "optimum" number of residues to change at one time during initial scanning of any new protein to identify important residues.

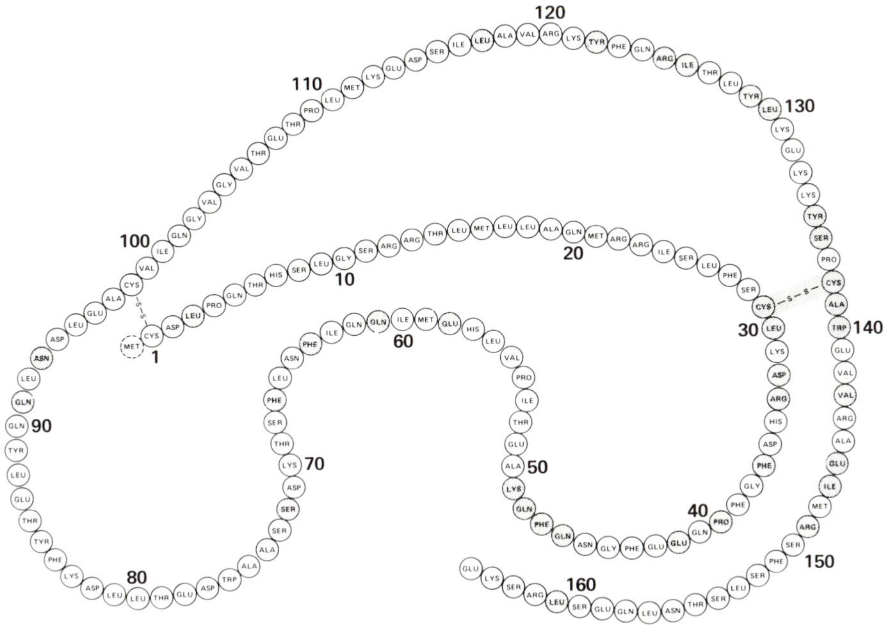

Fig. 14 IFN-α_2 sequence indicating residues conserved in all human IFN-α and IFN-β species.

Clusters of amino acids may be selected by a variety of criteria. In the first instance we chose the simplest, sequentially along the chain. Each group was chosen to fit into the structural elements described in one conformational model (Sternberg and Cohen, 1982). Following a well-established strategy used by synthetic chemists studying structure–activity relationships in small peptides (for a review see Rudinger, 1971), we planned first to replace all residues with alanine (except the one conserved alanine residue). This, in effect, attempted to identify critical amino acid side-chains by deleting them. Other coded amino acids could then be substituted at any position found to be important for activity.

This initial plan revealed technical limitations at almost every step. First, oligonucleotide purification and gene assembly proved difficult for some analogue genes. This may reflect secondary structure formation provoked by self-complementary GC dimers in closely spaced alanine codons. Next, we had no success in cloning genes for three analogues, [Ala^{41,46,47,48,49}]IFN-α_2, [Ala^{135,136,140}, Val^{139}]IFN-α_2 and [Ala^{143,146,147,149}]IFN-α_2. Finally, equivocal sequencing data were obtained for two analogue genes which did yield candidate clones, [Ala^{30,32,33,36,39}]IFN-α_2 and [Ala^{58,61,64,67,72,91,93}]IFN-α_2. Of the six initial target analogues, only [Ala^{117,122,125,126,129,130}]IFN-α_2 was successfully achieved. Overall, these results seem to indicate that smaller clusters, more widely-spaced changes or substitution with residues other than alanine should be selected. However, closely spaced alanine codons are not necessarily a problem, as was demonstrated by the successful cloning and expression of a gene for [Ala^{10-15}]IFN-α_2 (see Section VIII (A4)).

Lysate supernatants containing the analogue [$Ala^{117,122,125,126,129,130}$]IFN-$\alpha_2$ did not show antiviral activity and did not cross-react with NK2 or YOK monoclonal antibodies. However, minicells indicated that a new protein was being synthesized and immunoblotting demonstrated that this protein was recognized by a polyclonal antiserum raised against IFN-α_2. The six conserved residues changed in this analogue are found in one strand of the antiparallel β-sheet structure proposed in the conformational model. They lie between the region of residues 112–113, important for NK2-recognition (Section VIII (B1)), and the region around residue Cys138.

Three related analogues have been prepared in an attempt to define further the relative importance of these conserved residues. [$Ala^{122,125,126,129,130}$]IFN-$\alpha_2$ did not show antiviral activity and was not recognized by NK2. [$Ala^{129,130}$]IFN-α_2 was also antiviral inactive but did show some cross-reaction with NK2. However, it was not retained by and could not be purified on NK2-Sepharose. [$Ala^{125,126}$]IFN-α_2 was both antiviral active and NK2 cross-reactive (specific antiviral activity about 3×10^6 IU/mg; 5×10^8 NK2-IRMA U/mg). We conclude that conserved residues Arg125 and Ile126 cannot be essential for activity, but that loss of the side-chains from these two residues does lead to a fall in antiviral potency. Residues Tyr129 and Leu130 would be worthy of further investigation.

An analogue of a fusion protein of IFN-α_1 with the equivalent of a single Tyr122 to Gly change has been prepared by site-directed mutagenesis (Nisbet *et al.*, 1985). This showed less than 1% of the antiviral activity of the parent fusion protein (IFN-α_1 with nine additional amino acids at the *N*-terminus) on human cells but no significant loss of antiviral activity on primary bovine cells.

Site-directed mutagenesis has also been used to produce analogues of IFN-α_2 with single residue changes at conserved amino acids in positions 47 (Phe to Tyr, Ser or Cys), 48 (Gln to His) and 61 (Gln to Lys) (Valenzuela *et al.*, 1985). None of these changes had any effect on either antiviral or antiproliferative activity. This has prompted the suggestion (Nisbet *et al.*, 1985) that the cluster of conserved amino acids in the 28–80 section of α-IFNs may be relatively unimportant for biological activity. Further studies of our own do not support this speculative suggestion.

Following our initial, largely unsuccessful, attempts to scan all the conserved residues, we concentrated on the residues adjacent to the conserved cysteine in position 29. The analogue [$Ala^{30,32,33}$]IFN-α_2 proved inactive in all our bioassays on human cells, but was still recognized by NK2 and YOK (Table II) and was purified using NK2-Sepharose (Camble *et al.*, 1985, 1986). Both amino acid composition analysis and sequence analysis of the *N*-terminal 33 residues gave the expected changes relative to IFN-α_2. In collaboration with us, Fabrizio Marcucci and Edward De Maeyer have demonstrated that this analogue is also devoid of antiviral and antiproliferative activity on bovine MDBK cells. However, whereas the analogue does not inhibit the binding of radiolabelled IFN-α_2 to human WISH cells, it does compete for binding and can act as a competitive antagonist of the antiviral and antiproliferative effects of IFN-α_2 on MDBK cells (Marcucci and De Maeyer, 1986).

Conserved residues Leu30, Asp32 and Arg33 are found on the second strand of the proposed antiparallel β-sheet and roughly opposite conserved residues Tyr129 and Leu130 on the other strand discussed above. Continued recognition of [Ala^{30,32,33}]IFN-α_2 by two monoclonal antibodies with distinct epitope requirements and by the human IFN-α_2 receptor on bovine cells suggested that deletion of the three conserved amino acid side-chains had not led to major changes in the overall conformation of the protein. It seemed possible that one or more of these three side-chains was intimately involved in the production of a biological response. We prepared eight more analogues to explore the importance of each of the three residues (Camble *et al.*, 1986). No clone was identified expressing the ninth planned analogue, [Ala^{30}]IFN-α_2.

All eight single-residue-replacement analogues showed similar specific immunoradiometric reactivities, but they varied widely in their antiviral potencies on human cells (Table II). Conservative replacement of the hydrophobic Leu30 residue with Ile had no significant effect on antiviral activity. More drastic substitution with a hydrophilic but approximately isosteric Asn residue produced a 100-fold drop in specific antiviral activity. Nevertheless, conservation of a hydrophobic side-chain in position 30 clearly is not essential for biological activity. The carboxylic acid side-chain of Asp32 was extended in [Glu^{32}]IFN-α_2, neutralized in [Asn^{32}]IFN-α_2 and deleted in [Ala^{32}]IFN-α_2 with no effect on antiviral activity. Neither the size nor the charge of this conserved side-chain appears to be important, in isolation, for activity. Removing the side-chain of Arg33 in [Ala^{33}]IFN-α_2 produced at least a 1000-fold drop in specific antiviral activity. Even conservative substitution with lysine at this position produced a major fall in potency on human cells. Introduction of an extended unbranched but hydrophobic side-chain in [Met^{33}]IFN-α_2 destroyed any detectable antiviral activity on human cells.

Despite the wide variation in antiviral activities on human cells shown by these analogues, there was no indication of any significant separation of antiviral from antiproliferative activity (Table II). In every case the ratio of

TABLE II Specific Activities of Purified Conserved Residue Replacement Analogues

Analogue	Partial Sequence				Specific Activity (U/mg)			Antiproliferative activity (Antiviral U/ml for 50% inhibition)
	Position				IRMA		Antiviral	
	30	31	32	33	NK2	YOK	WISH	DAUDI
IFN-α_2	– Leu –	Lys –	Asp –	Arg –	2.5×10^9	7×10^6	2×10^8	5
[Ala^{30,32,33}]IFN-α_2	Ala		Ala	Ala	9.0×10^8	8×10^6	Inactive	Inactive
[Ile^{30}]IFN-α_2	Ile				1.5×10^9	N.D.	6×10^7	6
[Asn^{30}]IFN-α_2	Asn				1.5×10^9	1×10^7	5×10^5	4
[Ala^{32}]IFN-α_2			Ala		2.0×10^9	N.D.	4×10^8	4
[Glu^{32}]IFN-α_2			Glu		7.5×10^8	N.D.	2×10^8	4
[Asn^{32}]IFN-α_2			Asn		1.5×10^9	N.D.	7×10^7	4
[Ala^{33}]IFN-α_2				Ala	1.5×10^9	6×10^6	8×10^4	4
[Lys^{33}]IFN-α_2				Lys	1.0×10^9	5×10^6	3×10^5	5
[Met^{33}]IFN-α_2				Met	2.0×10^9	1×10^7	$<2 \times 10^{3}$[a]	None detected

[a] Limit of assay; no activity detected at highest concentrations used
N.D. not determined.

antiviral to antiproliferative activities remained almost unchanged. Although biological activity is very sensitive to changes at Arg33, even this residue cannot be considered essential for activity, for [Ala^{33}]IFN-α_2 still produces consistent low-level biological effects on human cells. It is only when this side-chain deletion is combined with other deletions in the neighbouring conserved residues Asp32 and Leu30 that a complete loss of activity is achieved. The strategy of replacing several amino acids at a time provided important structure–activity information not obviously available by altering amino acid residues one at a time. This became even more apparent when the antiviral activities of the eight single residue replacement analogues were measured on bovine MDBK cells (Marcucci and De Maeyer, unpublished data). Whereas [Ala^{30,32,33}]IFN-α_2 is devoid of antiviral activity on MDBK cells at concentrations 10^5–10^6 times higher than those required to show antiviral activity with IFN-α_2, all the single residue substitution analogues, including [Met^{33}]IFN-α_2, possessed high specific antiviral activities.

Overall, [Ala^{30,32,33}]IFN-α_2 demonstrates that, at least in combination, the integrity of the conserved side-chains of Leu30, Asp32 and Arg33 is critical for both binding and biological activity on human cells but is critical only for biological activity on bovine cells. Thus, at these three positions, the structural requirements for binding must be different for the cells used from the two species. The wide variation in antiviral activities of the single residue replacement analogues on human cells compared with their relative constancy on bovine cells suggests that, at these three positions, the structural requirements for biological activity may also be different for human WISH and bovine MDBK cells.

IX CONCLUSIONS AND PROSPECTS

Recombinant DNA technology has already had a significant impact on pharmaceutical research by revealing a wealth of sequence information on natural proteins of potential therapeutic value and by opening new avenues for the production of such natural proteins in the quantities required for clinical evaluation and use. In a second generation, the technology has now been extended to allow the preparation of sequence variants of natural proteins with residues deleted from the polypeptide chain or other genetically-coded amino acids added on to or substituted into the chain. Our own efforts, described in this review, have centred on evaluating the potential of synthetic genes to generate sequence analogues of IFN-α_2.

Looking back at the three strategic questions we took as objectives, we are convinced that the synthetic gene approach can produce target analogues with the throughput required to make progress in a protein structure–activity programme. The methodology is still being refined and is still far from routine, but in a two-and-a-half-year period we were able to examine over 100 sequence variants of IFN-α_2, some 60 of which are mentioned in this review. A particular advantage of synthetic genes is that multiple changes can be introduced simultaneously anywhere in the sequence.

With IFN-α_2, many analogues of diverse types proved sufficiently robust when prepared in *E. coli* that coherent structure–activity patterns were obtained without recourse to multi-step purification protocols or complex protein-folding procedures. Antibody reagents, however, do provide a simple one-step method of purification from crude bacterial lysate extracts to allow monitoring of heterogeneity and determination of specific activities in target-analogue-related proteins. We have demonstrated that up to ten residues can be removed from either end of the polypeptide chain and residues 10–15 and 98–114 can be replaced with completely unrelated amino acids with little change in biological activity. These results confirm that the Cys1–Cys98 disulphide bridge is not important for activity. Changes to the Cys29–Cys138 disulphide generally lead to a loss of biological activity, but we have shown, surprisingly, that significant activity is retained when both cysteine residues are replaced by serine. The integrity of either disulphide bridge is not required for cross-reactivity with the NK2-monoclonal antibody. However, the dipeptide sequence Lys112–Glu113 in IFN-α_2 does appear to make an important contribution to the epitope for this antibody. Perhaps the most exciting structure–activity outcome of this whole programme was the discovery that [$Ala^{30,32,33}$]IFN-α_2 can act as a competitive antagonist of the antiviral and antiproliferative effects of IFN-α_2 on bovine MDBK cells. The retention of antiviral activity in analogues with only one of these three conserved residues changed emphasizes how important structure–activity information may sometimes only be revealed by replacing several amino acids at a time.

Apart from some separation of antiviral from antiproliferative activity in IFN-α_2(4–155), none of our analogues has provided any real key to increased selectivity of action. That this can be achieved has been clearly demonstrated by the studies with IFN-αJ (Ortaldo *et al.*, 1984). Site-directed mutagenesis has been used to prepare a variant of IFN-αJ with the Phe115 residue replaced with Ser. Preliminary results indicate that this single change restored natural killer cell activity to IFN-αJ to a significant degree (Pestka *et al.*, 1985). We were also intrigued by this Phe115 residue in IFN-αJ, since a serine residue occurs at this position in all other human IFN-α species and in IFN-β. We prepared [Phe^{115}]IFN-α_2, but this analogue still showed good natural killer-cell-stimulating activity.

There is still much work to be done in defining the structural correlates of biological activity in IFN-α. The results that have emerged from our own and other studies already provide optimism that the use of recombinant DNA techniques to manipulate protein structures can lead to analogues with new and interesting biological profiles. Once a limited number of amino acid residues of particular importance has been identified, the 20 genetically-coded L-amino acids provide only a limited selection of structural variations. To extend protein structure–activity studies into analogues with other structural features will require a third-generation exploitation of recombinant DNA. Protein modification or protein semi-synthesis techniques will have to be applied to an initial biosynthetic product. Both approaches might be facilitated by appropriate tailoring of the parent protein produced in bacteria. For example, subsequent protein semi-synthesis (for a review see Offord, 1980) could be assisted if inconvenient cleavage sites present in the parent protein are eliminated by substitution with other amino acids still compatible with retention of biological activity. Thus, as described earlier (Section VIII (C)), we have prepared the analogue in which all five methionines in IFN-α_2 are replaced with leucines. New methionine residues could now be introduced into this analogue at any desired positions in the chain. The resulting bacterial product on treatment with cyanogen bromide should then generate fragments specifically designed for convenient semi-synthetic re-assembly around a chemically synthesized segment containing non-coded structural elements.

ACKNOWLEDGEMENTS

The work described in this review would not have been possible without considerable technical assistance. We wish to thank Gill Fossdyke and Dave Holland for oligonucleotide synthesis; April Greene and Clive Newton for gene synthesis; Clive Newton for gene cloning; Angela Cunningham, April Greene and Phil Trueman for DNA sequencing; Ian Taylor and John Spedding for fermentation work; Nigel Petter and Phil Trueman for protein isolation, characterization and immunoradiometric assays; Lesley Farrow and Doug Paterson for protein HPLC and anti-2 polyclonal antisera; Nigel Faulkner and Margaret Bowen for bioassays; and finally Anne Greenslade for preparing this manuscript.

REFERENCES

Ackerman, S. K., Zur Nedden, D., Heintzelman, M., Hunkapiller, M. and Zoon, K. C. (1984). *Proc. Natl. Acad. Sci. USA* **81**, 1045–1047.
Aguet, M. and Blanchard, B. (1981). *Virology* **115**, 249–261.
Allen, G. and Fantes, K. H. (1980) *Nature (London)* **287**, 408–411.

Arenzana-Seisdedos, F. and Virelizier, J. L. (1983). *Eur. J. Immunol.* **13**, 437–440.

Arnheiter, H., Ohno, M., Smith, M., Gutte, B. and Zoon, K. C. (1983). *Proc. Natl. Acad. Sci. USA* **80**, 2539–2543.

Bidlingmeyer, B. A., Cohen, S. A. and Tarvin, T. L. (1984). *J. Chromatography* **336**, 93–104.

Boraschi, D., Censini, S. and Tagliabue, A. (1984). *J. Immunol.* **133**, 764–768.

Branca, A. A. and Baglioni, C. (1981). *Nature (London)* **294**, 768–770.

Camble, R., Edge, M. D. and Moore, V. E. (1985). *In* "Peptides; Structure and Function". Proceedings 9th American Peptide Symposium Toronto (C. M. Deber, V. J. Hruby and K. D. Kopple, eds.). pp. 375–384. Pierce Chemical Co., Rockford, Ill.

Camble, R., Petter, N. N., Trueman, P., Newton, C. R., Carr, F. J., Hockney, R. C., Moore, V. E., Greene, A. R., Holland, D. and Edge, M. D. (1986). *Biochem. Biophys. Res. Commun.* **134**, 1404–1411.

Chang, N. T., Kung, H.-F. and Pestka, S. (1983). *Arch. Biochem. Biophys.* **221**, 585–589.

Content, J. and Derynck, R. (1983). *La Récherche* **14**, 232–235.

DeGrado, W. F., Wasserman, Z. R. and Chowdhry, V. (1982). *Nature (London)* **300**, 379–381.

De Maeyer, E., Skup, D., Prasad, K. S. N., De Maeyer-Guignard, J., Williams, B., Meacock, P., Sharpe, G., Pioli, D., Hennam, J., Schuch, W. and Atherton, K. (1982). *Proc. Natl Acad. Sci. USA* **79**, 4256–4259.

Derynck, R., Gray, P. W., Yelverton, E., Leung, D. W., Shepard, H. M., Lawn, R. M., Ullrich, A., Najarian, R., Pennica, D., Hagie, F. E., Hitzeman, R. A., Sherwood, P. J., Levinson, A. D. and Goeddel, D. V. (1982). *In* "From Gene to Protein: Translation into Biotechnology", pp. 249–262. Academic Press, New York.

Edge, M. D. and Camble, R. (1984). *In* "Biotechnology and Genetic Engineering Reviews" (G. E. Russell, ed.), vol. 2, pp. 215–252. Intercept, UK.

Edge, M. D., Greene, A. R., Heathcliffe, G. R., Meacock, P. A., Schuch, W., Scanlon, D. B., Atkinson, T. C., Newton, C. R. and Markham, A. F. (1981). *Nature (London)* **292**, 756–762.

Edge, M. D., Greene, A. R., Heathcliffe, G. R., Moore, V. E., Faulkner, N. J., Camble, R., Petter, N. N., Trueman, P., Schuch. W., Hennam, J., Atkinson, T. C., Newton, C. R. and Markham, A. F. (1983). *Nucleic Acids Res.* **11**, 6419–6435.

Evinger, M., Rubinstein, M. and Pestka, S. (1981). *Arch. Biochem. Biophys.* **210**, 319–329.

Felix, A. M., Heimer, E. P., Lamdros, T. J., Swistok, J., Tarnowski, S. J. and Wang, C. T. (1985). *J. Chromatography* **327**, 359–368.

Frank, R., Heikens, W., Heisterberg-Moutsis, G. and Bloecker, H. (1983). *Nucleic Acids Res.* **11**, 4365–4377.

Franke, A. E., Shepard, H. M., Houck, C. M., Leung, D. W., Goeddel, D. V. and Lawn, R. M. (1982). *DNA* **1**, 223–230.

Gait, M. J. and Sheppard, R. C. (1977). *Nucleic Acids Res.* **4**, 1135–1158.

Gait, M. J., Singh, M., Sheppard, R. C., Edge, M. D., Greene, A. R., Heathcliffe, G. R., Atkinson, T. C., Newton, C. R. and Markham, A. F. (1980). *Nucleic Acids Res.* **8**, 1081–1096.

Gait, M. J., Matthes, H. W. D., Singh, M. and Titmas, R. C. (1982). *J. Chem. Soc., Chem. Commun.* 37–40.

Goeddel, D. V., Leung, D. W., Dull, T. J., Gross, M., Lawn, R. M., McCandliss, R., Seeburg, P. H., Ullrich, A., Yelverton, E. and Gray, P. W. (1981). *Nature (London)* **290**, 20–26.

Gray, P. W. and Goeddel, D. V. (1982). *Nature (London)* **298**, 859–863.

Hamilton, J. A., Zabriskie, J. D., Lachman, L. B. and Chen, Y. S. (1982). *J. Exp. Med.* **155**, 1702–1718.

Hanahan, D. (1983). *J. Mol. Biol.* **166**, 557–580.

Hayden, F. G., Mills, S. E. and Johns, M. E. (1983). *J. Infect. Dis.* **148**, 914–921.

Hayes, T. (1980). *Biochem. Biophys. Res. Commun.* **95**, 872–879.

Hunkapiller, M. W. and Hood, L. E. (1983). *Science* **219**, 650–659.

Joshi, A. R., Sarkar, F. H. and Gupta, S. L. (1982). *J. Biol. Chem.* **257**, 13884–13887.

Levy, W. P., Rubinstein, M., Shively, J., Del Valle, U., Lai, C.-Y., Moschera, J., Brink, L., Gerber, L., Stein, S. and Pestka, S. (1981). *Proc. Natl Acad. Sci. USA* **78**, 6186–6190.

Lydon, N. B., Favre, C., Bove, S., Neyret, O., Benureau, S., Levine, A. M., Seelig, G. F., Nagabhushan, L, and Trotta, P. P. (1985). *Biochemistry* **24**, 4131–4141.

Mantei, N., Schwarzstein, M., Streuli, M., Panem, S., Nagata, S. and Weissmann, C. (1980). *Gene* **10**, 1–10.

Marcucci, F. and De Maeyer, E. (1986). *Biochem. Biophys. Res. Commun.* **134**, 1412–1418.

Markham, A. F., Edge, M. D., Atkinson, T. C., Greene, A. R., Heathcliffe, G. R., Newton, C. R. and Scanlon, D. (1980). *Nucleic Acids Res.* **8**, 5193–5205.

Marx, J. L. (1983) *Science* **221**, 1362–1364.

Maury, C. P. J., Enholm, E. and Teppo, A. M. (1983). *New Engl. J. Med.* **309**, 1060.

Merlin, G., Falcoff, E. and Aguet, M. (1985). *J. Gen. Virol.* **66**, 1149–1152.

Merrifield, R. B. (1983). *In* "Peptides: Structure and Function". Proceedings 8th American Peptide Symposium (V. J. Hruby and D. H. Rich, eds.). pp. 34–44. Pierce Chemical Co., Rockford, Ill.

Mizel, S. B., Dayer, J. M., Krane, S. M. and Mergenhangen, S. E. (1981). *Proc. Natl Acad. Sci. USA* **78**, 2474–2477.

Morehead, H., Johnston, P. D. and Wetzel, R. (1984). *Biochemistry* **23**, 2500–2507.

Nagata, S., Mantei, N. and Weissmann, C. (1980). *Nature (London)* **287**, 401–408.

Newton, C. R., Greene, A. R., Heathcliffe, G. R., Atkinson, T. C., Holland, D., Markham, A. F. and Edge, M. D. (1983). *Anal. Biochem.* **129**, 22–30.

Nisbet, I. T., Beilharz, M. W., Hertzog, P. J., Tymms, M. J. and Linnane, A. W. (1985). *Biochem. Int.* **11**, 301–309.

Offord, R. E. (1980). "Semisynthetic Proteins". Wiley, Chichester, New York, Brisbane, Toronto.

Ortaldo, J. R., Herberman, R. B., Harvey, C., Osheroff, P., Pan, Y. C. E., Kelder, B. and Pestka, S. (1984). *Proc. Natl Acad. Sci. USA* **81**, 4926–4929.

Pestka, S., Kelder, B., Tarnowski, D. K. and Tarnowski, S. J. (1983). *Anal. Biochem.* **132**, 328–333.

Pestka, S., Labdon, J. E., Rashidbaigi, A., Liu, X-Y., Langer, J. A., Ortaldo, J. R., Herberman, R. B. and Jung, V. (1985). *In* "The Biology of the Interferon System 1984" (H. Kirchner and H. Schellekens, eds.), pp. 3–11. Elsevier/North Holland, Amsterdam.

Rudinger, J. (1971). *In* "Drug Design" (E. J. Ariens, ed.), vol. 2, pp. 319–419. Academic Press, New York.

Schmidt, J. A., Mizel, S. B. and Green, I. (1981). *Fed. Proc.* **40**, 1084.

Scott, G. M., Ward, R. J., Wright, D. J., Robinson, J. A., Onwubalili, J. K. and Gauci, C. L. (1983). *Antimicrob. Agents Chemother.* **23**, 589–592.

Shepard, H. M., Leung, D., Stebbing, N. and Goeddel, D. V. (1981). *Nature (London)* **294**, 563–565.

Sternberg, M. J. E. and Cohen, F. E. (1982). *Int. J. Biol. Macromol.* **4**, 137–144.

Streuli, M., Nagata, S. and Weissmann, C. (1980). *Science* **209**, 1343–1347.

Streuli, M., Hall, A., Boll, W., Stewart, W. E., Nagata, S. and Weissmann, C. (1981). *Proc. Natl Acad. Sci. USA* **78**, 2848–2852.

Taniguchi, T., Mantei, N., Schwarzstein, M., Nagata, S., Muramatsu, M. and Weissmann, C. (1980). *Nature* **285**, 547–549.

Towbin, H. and Gordon, J. (1984). *J. Immunol. Methods* **72**, 313–340.

Traub, A., Feinstein, S., Grosfeld, H., Payess, B., Lazar, A., Reuveny, S. and Mizrahi, A. (1981). *J. Interferon Res.* **1**, 571–579.

Trown, P. W., Heimer, E. P., Felix, A. M. and Bohoslawec, O. (1985). In "Biology of the Interferon System" (H. Kirchner and H. Schellekens, eds.), pp. 69–76. Elsevier, Amsterdam.

Valenzuela, D., Weber, H. and Weissmann, C. (1985) *Nature (London)* **313**, 698–700.

Wallace, R. B., Johnson, M. J., Suggs, S. V., Miyoshi, K., Bhatt, R. and Itakura, K. (1981). *Gene* **16**, 21–26.

Weissmann, C. (1981). European Patent Application 32,134, p. 74.

Weissmann, C., Nagata, S., Boll, W., Fountoulakis, M., Fujisawa, A., Fujisawa, J.-I., Haynes, J., Henco, K., Mantei, N., Ragg, H., Schein, C., Schmid, J., Shaw, G., Streuli, M., Taira, H., Todokoro, K. and Weidle, U. (1982). *Phil. Trans. R. Soc. London* **B299**, 7–28.

Wetzel, R. (1981). *Nature (London)* **289**, 606–607.

Wetzel, R., Perry, L. J., Estell, D. A., Lin, N., Levine, H. L., Slinker, B., Fields, F., Ross., M. J. and Shively, J. (1981). *J. Interferon. Res.* **1**, 381–390.

Wetzel, R., Levine, H. L., Estell, D. A., Shire, S., Finer-Moore, J., Stroud, R. M. and Bewley, T. A. (1982). *In* "Chemistry and Biology of Interferons: Relationship to Therapeutics" (T. Merigan, R. Friedman and C. F. Cox, eds.), pp. 365–376. Academic Press, New York.

Wetzel, R., Johnston, P. D. and Czarnlecki, C. W. (1983). In "Biology of the Interferon System" (E. De Maeyer and H. Schellekens, eds.), pp. 101–112. Elsevier, Amsterdam.

Windass, J. D., Newton, C. R., De Maeyer-Guignard, J., Moore, V. E., Markham, A. F. and Edge, M. D. (1982). *Nucleic Acids Res.* **10**, 6639–6657.

Wray, W., Boulikas, T., Wray, V. P. and Hancock, R. (1981). *Anal. Biochem.* **118**, 197–203.

Yonehara, S., Yonehara-Takahashi, M. and Ishii, A. (1983). *J. Virol.* **45**, 1168–1171.

Zav'yalov, V. P. and Denesyuk, A. I. (1982). *Immunol. lett.* **4**, 7–14.

Zoon, K. C. and Wetzel, R. (1984). *In* "Handbook of Experimental Pharmacology" (P. E. Crane and W. A. Carter, eds.), vol. 71 pp. 79–100. Springer-Verlag, Berlin.

Interferon and Major Histocompatibility Complex Genes: A Model to Analyse Eukaryotic Gene Regulation?

FRÉDÉRIC M. ROSA*, MADELEINE M. COCHET[†] AND MARC FELLOUS*

* *Immunogénétique Humaine, Unité INSERM 276, Institut Pasteur, 25 rue du Docteur Roux, 75724 Paris Cedex 15.*
[†] *Biologie Moléculaire du Gène, Unité INSERM 277, Institut Pasteur, 25 rue du Docteur Roux, 75724 Paris Cedex 15.*

INTERFERON 7
ISBN 0 12 302256 8

Major histocompatibility complex (MHC) is a multigene family, located on chromosome 6 in man or 17 in the mouse, that controls graft rejection in mammals. More generally, the MHC is involved in the control of various immune reactions such as T cell recognition, antigen presentation, etc. (Ploegh *et al.*, 1981). This multigene family is subdivided into three classes of genes. Class III genes encode for complement components. Class I and class II genes encode for cell surface glycoproteins. Class I genes (class II) will be referred to as HLA-A, B, C in man (HLA-DR, DP, DQ) or H-2D, K, L in mouse (H-2IA, IE).

I EFFECT OF IFN ON MHC EXPRESSION

When human cells are treated by human interferon, regardless of its type, there is an increase of the level of HLA-A, B, C antigens on the cell surface. Following IFN-α, -β or -γ treatment from 10 U/ml to 2×10^3 U/ml, the increase of HLA class I antigens on human cells is rapid (detectable after one hour), stable for at least 24 hours and dramatic (from 2 to 10 times the initial level present at the surface of untreated cells).

The enhancement of HLA class I cell surface antigens upon IFN treatment is preceded by an increase in HLA class I protein synthesis. A typical enhancement of HLA class I protein synthesis upon IFN-γ treatment of human T cell line MOLT4 cells is presented in Fig. 1. The protein synthesis of both HLA heavy chains and β_2 microglobulin (which is necessary for the cell surface expression of HLA class I molecules) display a 3- to 5-fold increase after IFN treatment for 24 or 48 hours.

Northern blot analysis of mRNA encoding HLA class I heavy chains has shown that IFN treatment increases the steady state level of HLA-A, -B, -C mRNA in every cell type studied (Fellous *et al.*, 1982a). For instance, treatment of human lymphoblastoid cell line Ramos with IFN-α, -β or-γ (Fig. 2) increased HLA class I mRNA in a 4–6 fold ratio.

The effect of IFN on MHC cell surface antigens was initially described on mouse L1210 cells by Gresser *et al.* (Lindahl *et al.*, 1973). Since then, several reports have confirmed these results (Table I) in several species including man.

The enhancement of MHC class I antigens upon IFN treatment has been shown *in vitro* as well as *in vivo* (Table I). With the exception of IFN-resistant cell lines, most of the cells studied express more MHC class I antigens when they have been incubated in the presence of IFN. In particular, human melanoma cell lines and embryonic fibroblasts (Fig. 3) synthesize more HLA, -A, -B, -C antigens when they are treated with IFN-α, -β or -γ.

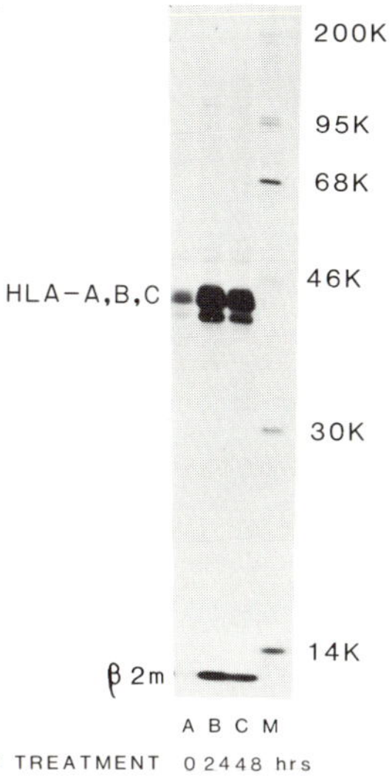

Fig. 1. Effect of IFN-γ on MOLT 4 cells. MOLT 4 cells were treated for 24 or 48 hours with 500 U/ml recombinant IFN-γ and pulse-labelled with ^{35}S methionine lysed with TX 114 (Rosa *et al.*, 1983a) and immunoprecipitated (Rosa *et al.*, 1983a) with anti-HLA monoclonal antibody B.9.12.1 (gift from Dr Malissen). The precipitate was processed as described (Rosa *et al.*, 1983a) on an SDS-PAGE and exposed to XAR-5 film. A, no treatment; B, IFN-γ for 24 hours; C, IFN-γ for 48 hours; M, molecular weight markers. Reprinted from the *Annales de l'Institute Pasteur*, with permission.

Does IFN act on other cell surface antigens?

The increase in cell surface antigens, protein synthesis or mRNA levels upon IFN treatment is not restricted to HLA-A, -B, -C, antigens. The synthesis of β2m which is associated with HLA heavy chain in HLA class I antigens, is also increased. A detailed review on the effect of IFN cell surface antigens has been recently published (Gresser, 1983).

The case of HLA class II antigens is more peculiar and has for a long time been controversial (Table I). However, HLA-DR protein synthesis and mRNA levels are increased upon IFN treatment in melanoma cells, particularly when IFN-γ is used (Fig. 3). In BEL melanoma cells, IFN-γ enhances both HLA-DRα and -β synthesis and mRNA levels by at least 10-fold (Rosa *et al.*, 1983a). The effect of IFN on MHC antigens appears to be a common property of IFN classes. In particular IFN-γ as well as IFN-α or -β are able to stimulate class I as well as class II MHC gene activity.

However, type I and type II IFN differ from each other in the following respects.

(1) IFN-γ, in contrast to IFN-α or -β, enhances MHC class I gene products at very low concentrations (0.1 or 0.01 antiviral units/ml), whereas

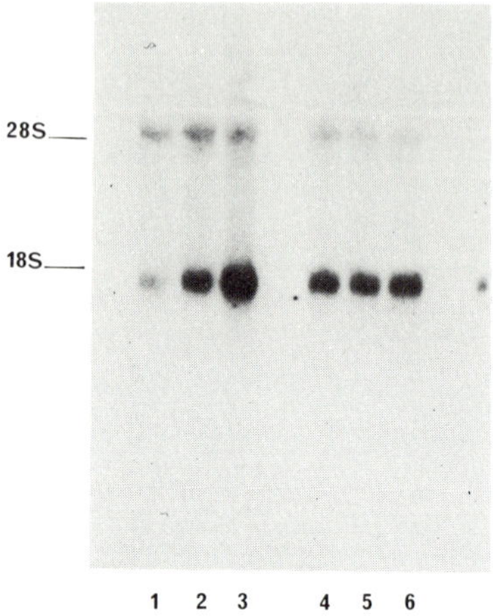

Fig. 2 Effect of IFN-α and -β on HLA mRNA levels in Ramos lymphoid cells. PolyA + RNA were extracted from treated or untreated cells and analysed by Northern blotting using an HLA-A, B, C cDNA probe (Fellous *et al.*, 1982a). HLA mRNA migrates just below the 18S ribosomal RNA. 1, 2, 3: RAMOS mRNA. 4, 5, 6: Namalwa mRNA. 1, 4: no treatment. 2, 5: IFN-α at 500 U/ml for 24 hours. 3, 6: IFN-β at 500 U/ml for 24 hours.

IFN type I must be present in the medium at concentrations of at least 10 U/ml to produce a similar effect on MHC class I gene products (Wallach *et al.*, 1982). The effect of IFN-γ on MHC class I antigens can be seen at concentrations that do not promote antiviral resistance.

(2) Only IFN-γ is able significantly to increase MHC class II gene products (Table I).

For both these reasons, it is now assumed that IFN-γ with several other lymphokines may play a major role in MHC regulation in addition to direct antiviral protection.

Is IFN the factor responsible?

Many of the experiments referred to above have been performed with partially purified or highly purified preparations of IFNs. These preparations, particularly IFN-γ preparations, may have been contaminated by molecules other than IFN that could have been responsible for MHC regulation.

If we cannot exclude the presence in IFN preparations of molecules different from IFN, then IFN itself appears able to regulate MHC antigens expression for the following reasons: Firstly, it is possible to prevent MHC class I or class II glycoprotein synthesis enhancement upon IFN-γ treatment by incubating IFN-γ with a monoclonal antibody that blocks IFN-γ activity (Rosa *et al.*, 1983a). Similar results were obtained in our laboratory with

TABLE I (Abbreviations: CS = Cell Surface, NP = Neosynthesized proteins)

Authors	MHC class, species	Cells	Type and source of IFN	Levels of analysis: CS	NP	mRNA
Lindahl *et al.*, 1973 (1)	I Mouse	Lymphoid	IFN-α, β	+		
Heron *et al.*, 1978 (2)	I Man	Peripheral blood lymphocytes (PBL)	IFN-α	+		
Fellous *et al.*, 1978 (3)	I Man	PBL, lymphoid cell lines	IFN-α	+		
Wallach *et al.*, 1982 (4)	I Man	Lymphoid and fibroblastic cell lines	Purified IFN-α, β, γ Recombinant IFN-γ	+	+	+
Basham *et al.*, 1982 (5)	I Man	Melanomas	Purified IFN-β, γ		+	
Burrone and Milstein 1982 (6)	I Man	T cell line MOLT 4	Purified IFN-α	+	+	+
Fellous *et al.*, 1982 (7)	I, II Man	Lymphoid and fibroblastic cell lines	Purified IFN-α, β	+	negative for class II	+
Pober *et al.*, 1983 (8)	II Man	Human vascular endothelial fibroblasts (HUVE)	"ConA supernatant" Recombinant IFN-γ	+		
Steeg *et al.*, 1982 (9)	II Mouse	Macrophage cell line	"ConA supernatant" purified IFN-γ	+		
Wong *et al.*, 1982 (10)	II Mouse	Mast cell progenitors	"PHA supernatant"	+		
Rosa *et al.*, 1983 (11)	I, II Man	Lymphoid and melanoma cell lines	Purified IFN-α, β, γ	+	+	+
Hirsch *et al.*, 1983 (12)	II Mouse	Brain astrocytes	Purified IFN-γ	+		
Basham *et al.*, 1983 (13)	II Man	Macrophage, melanoma cell lines	Recombinant IFN-α, γ	+	+	
Virelizier *et al.*, 1984 (14)	II Man	Monocytic cell lines	Recombinant IFN-α, γ Purified IFN-$\alpha\gamma$	+		
Wong *et al.*, 1984 (15)	I, II Mouse	B Lymphoid cells, macrophages	Recombinant IFN-α_2, γ	+		
Nakamura *et al.*, 1984 (16)	II Mouse	Macrophage cell line	Recombinant IFN-γ			+
Pober *et al.*, 1983 (17)	II Man	HUVE, human skin fibroblasts	Recombinant IFN-α_2, β, γ	+	+ recognition by CTL	
Dolei *et al.*, 1981 (18)	II Man	Lymphoid cell lines	Purified IFN-α, β, γ	+		

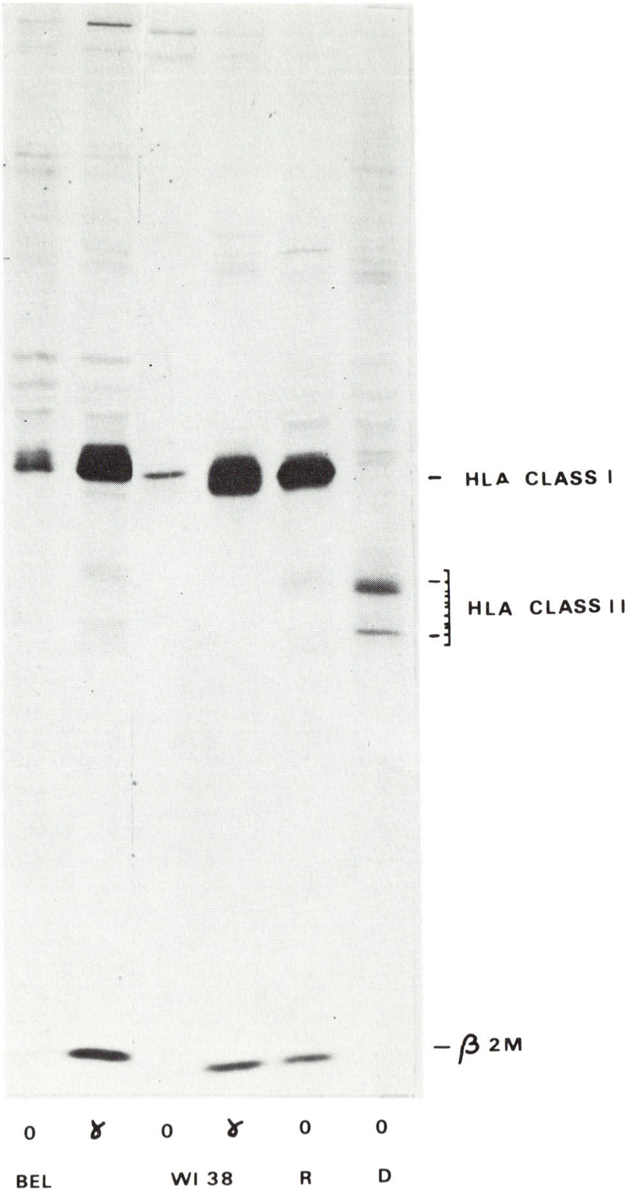

Fig. 3 Effect of IFN-β and -γ on class II antigens synthesis. IFN-treated cells were labelled and analysed as described in Fig. 1. BEL: melanoma. WI38: embryonic pulmonary fibroblast. R: Raji lymphoblastoid cell line. D: Daudi lymphoblastoid cell line. O: No treatment. γ: IFN-γ at 500 U/ml for 24 hours.

mAb directed against IFN-α or -β. Secondly it has been shown independently by different laboratories that recombinant IFN-α, -β or -γ are able to regulate MHC genes (Table I) with very similar effect. We do not exclude the possibility that other lymphokines produced by conA-stimulated lymphocytes (such as BCGF1) can regulate MHC antigen expression.

However, the effect of IFN on MHC antigens raises several issues that we will analyse in following sections.

How are IFNs able to regulate independent genes?

IFN-α, -β and -γ are able to regulate *HLA-A, B, C, HLA-DR* genes located on chromosome 6, and β2m, which is located on human chromosome 15. Even if parts of these genes are genetically linked, they behave as different genes. If they are coordinately regulated by the same factors, one might assume they share signals in common.

Is MHC antigen expression regulated by molecules other than IFN?

For a long time, IFN was the only biological molecule known to be able to regulate MHC antigen expression. Recently, B cell growth Factor 1 (BCGF1) has been shown to increase cell surface expression of MHC class II antigens on resting murine B cells (Le Meur *et al.*, 1985). The mechanism of BCGF or prostaglandin is not known so far.

Is the IFN-directed enhancement of class I and class II antigens a general phenomenon?

The IFN-directed enhancement of MHC class I and class II antigens has been observed on many cell types *in vivo* and *in vitro*. Our interest in the field, however, was complicated by a surprising finding. When analysing the effect of IFN on MHC cell surface antigens of many cell lines, we found cell lines sensitive to the effect of IFN-γ on class I but not class II cell surface antigens. IFN-γ was not able to increase HLA-DR antigens on Burkitt-lymphoma-derived cell lines. Furthermore, different cell lines of a common tissue type, melanoma for instance, were shown to respond differently to IFN-γ (class II cell surface antigens enhancement). Some melanomas appeared to be 'sensitive' to the effect of IFN-γ on HLA-DR cell surface antigens, whereas others were not (Rosa *et al.*, 1983a). Such a finding was also described independently by another laboratory (Houghton *et al.*, 1984).

When we analysed the effect of IFN-γ on the HLA-DR mRNA steady state level, we found that in every cell type studied that spontaneously express MHC class II genes, IFN-γ was able to increase HLA class II mRNA. These results are summarized in Table II. In 5 different human T cell lines studied

TABLE II Effect of IFN-γ on HLA Class II Gene Expression

	Endogenous class II level			
	Human melanoma cell lines		B-cell lines	T-cell lines
	High	Low	High	None
IFN-γ-induced level membrane	–	↑↑	–	–
Neosynthesized proteins	↑	↑↑	–	–
mRNA	↑↑	↑↑	↑↑	–

(–: no effect, ↑: increase).

(MOLT4, KE37, 1301, CEMT, HPB-ALL), no appearance of an HLA-DR product was observed after IFN-γ treatment despite their response to IFN-γ for HLA class I molecules. In 10 different human B cell lines, the effect of IFN-γ was always detected at the mRNA level, but a very weak effect or no effect was observed at the level of HLA class II molecules at the cytoplasmic or cell surface level. In a human melanoma cell line with low expression of the HLA class II molecules, IFN-γ greatly enhanced HLA-DR gene expression at the three levels analysed. However, in melanoma cell lines that are high expressors for HLA class II molecules the effect of IFN-γ was only observed at the mRNA level.

We do not know how to interpret these differences at present. Clearly, a mRNA study must be carried out to define a cell line "sensitive" or "resistant" to interferon. However, IFN has allowed us to describe several steps where HLA class II expression can be regulated.

Step 1. The mRNA level observed in T cell lines.
Step 2. The translational level observed in B cell lines.
Step 3. The post-translational level observed in high-expression melanoma cell lines.

Do IFNs regulate genes other than MHC *genes?*

IFNs have been shown to increase the level of many different proteins or mRNA in human and mouse cells (Gresser, 1983). The identity of some of these IFN-regulated proteins is known: tubulin (Fellous *et al.*, 1982b), methallothionein (Friedman and Stark, 1985), β_2 microglobulin (Wallach *et al.*, 1982). However, the majority of IFN-regulated proteins are not yet known. Meanwhile, the effect of IFN on gene regulation is relatively specific: in interferon-treated cells, there are no significant changes in overall mRNA or protein content. Furthermore, some proteins or mRNA have been shown to be unaffected by IFN treatment: actin (Fellous *et al.*, 1982b), Thy-1 antigen (Gresser, 1983), and some are decreased upon IFN treatment: *myc* oncogene (Jonak and Knight, 1984) and transferrin receptor (Besançon and Bourgeade, 1985).

Does IFN act qualitatively on MHC cell surface antigens?

Apart from the enhancement of antigen molecules present at the cell surface, IFN could modify the structure and/or environment of these antigens into the cell membrane. Such additional effects might explain the discrepancy we observed between the enhancement of HLA class II mRNA and corresponding cell surface antigens levels in cells treated with IFN-α. For instance, IFN might have affected the stability of HLA class II antigens. Pulse chase experiments performed in our laboratory contradicted this hypothesis. On the other hand, IFN could have affected cell membrane fluidity, thus preventing new molecules from entering the cell membrane. We have studied the effect of murine IFN on membrane fluidity of HLA-transformed L cells (P. Le Bouteiller, Z. Mishal and M. Fellous, personal communication). Fluidity of plasma membrane was studied in whole cells using fluorescence polarization with the fluorescent probe 1, 6-diphenyl-1,3,5-hexatriene (Esko *et al.*, 1977). These measurements reflected the fluidity in the surface membrane. Fluidity, the reciprocal of viscosity, is proportional to the molecular free volume and inversely proportional to the packing density of the fluid volume (Shinitzky and Henkart 1980). After IFN treatment, transformed L cells had greater fluidity, which means lower viscosity of the cell membrane. This effect is temperature-dependent.

II IFN AND INDUCTION OF SILENT GENES

Until recently, it was not clear whether IFN was able to induce the *de novo* synthesis of MHC gene products which are not spontaneously expressed. In particular, we were unable to induce synthesis of HLA-DR antigens in several human T-cell lines tested (Rosa *et al.*, 1983a). We postulated that IFN had to be regarded as an "amplifier' rather than as a real inducer.

A Induction of HLA Class I Antigens in Human K562 Cell Line

In order to re-investigate this hypothesis, we studied the effect of IFN on several clones from human erythroleukemic cell line K562, which is lacking class I as well as class II MHC gene expression (Sutherland *et al.*, 1985). Using highly purified IFN-α and -β or recombinant IFN-β or -γ, we have

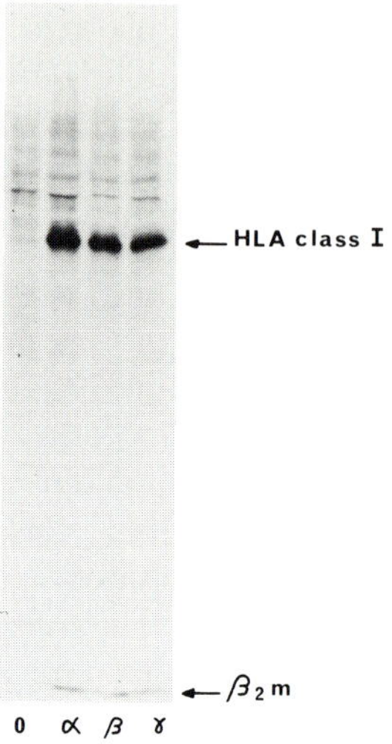

Fig. 4. Induction of HLA class I antigens in K562 upon IFN treatment. Following an overnight incubation with IFN-α, -β, -γ K562 cells were pulse-labelled, lysed and immunoprecipitated as described in Fig. 1. Reprinted from the *Annales de l'Institut Pasteur*, with permission.

demonstrated that IFN can induce cell surface expression of class I MHC antigen in K562. Immunoprecipitation carried out on an IFN-γ-treated K562 cell line pulse-labelled with ^{35}S-methionine (Fig. 4) shows the *de novo* induction of synthesis of HLA class I protein upon IFN treatment. We have also demonstrated that IFN can induce the appearance of class I MHC mRNA in K562. However, all our attempts to induce HLA class II molecules in K562 remained unsuccessful (Sutherland *et al.*, 1985) in mRNA and cell surface protein assays.

B Induction of HLA Class II Gene Expression

We also investigated the inducibility of HLA class II gene products upon IFN-γ treatment of non-expressing cells. Immunoprecipitation performed on several human skin fibroblast cell lines clearly shows (Fig. 5) the *de novo* induction of HLA-DR synthesis in these cells upon IFN-γ but not IFN-β treatment. These data confirmed the results described by Pober *et al.* concerning the inducibility of HLA-DR antigens and synthesis on human skin fibroblasts and human vascular endothelial fibroblasts (Pober *et al.*, 1983). Northern blots carried out using an HLA-DRα cDNA probe confirmed that IFN-γ can induce the appearance of HLA-DRα in several skin fibroblasts (Rosa *et al.*, 1985).

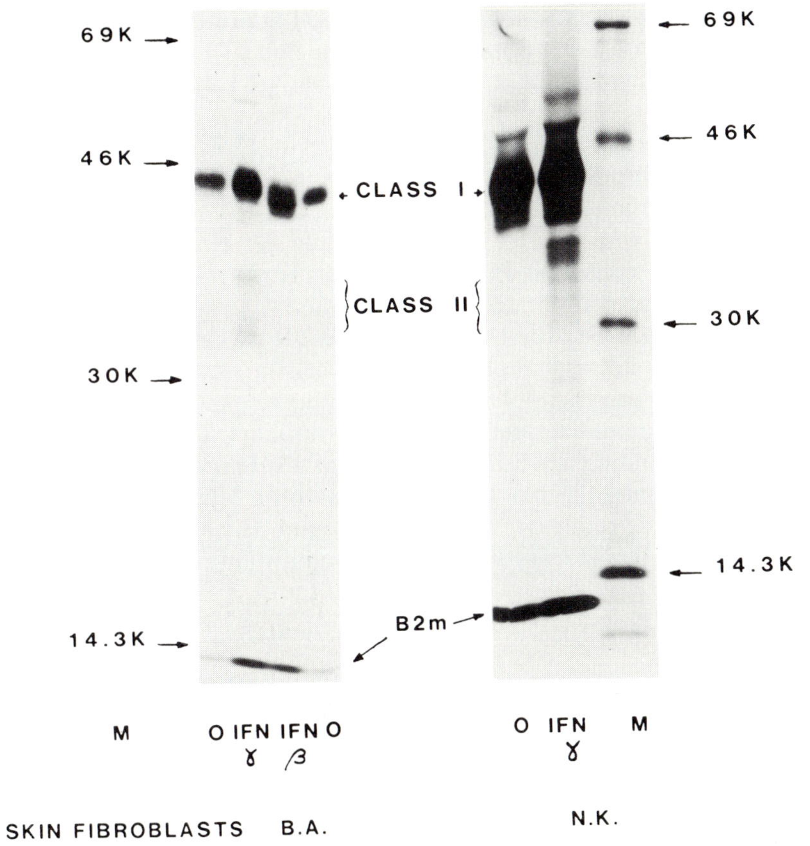

Fig. 5 Induction of HLA-DR antigens in human skin fibroblasts A and NK upon IFN-γ treatment. Following IFN treatment, human skin fibroblasts were analysed as in Fig. 1, except that immunoprecipitation was carried out with B 9.12.1 and V. 1.15.C (monoclonal antibody against HLA-DR, provided by Dr Pious). Reprinted from the *Annales de l'Institut Pasteur*, with permission.

IFN-γ has been shown to induce HLA class II gene expression on myelo-monocytic cell lines HL60 (Koeffler *et al.*, 1984), U937 (Virelizier *et al.*, 1984) or in astrocytes (Hirsch *et al.*, 1983). Different set of HLA class II genes appears to be regulated unequally by IFN-γ in HL60 on human skin fibroblasts. HLA-DQ gene expression is poorly induced in human skin fibroblasts upon IFN-γ treatment. HLA-DQ gene expression is not induced to detectable levels in HL60. Quite surprisingly, we failed to induce HLA-DR gene products in WI38, an embryonic pulmonary fibroblast cell line, or bone-marrow-derived human fibroblast SV80. Therefore, the inducibility of class II MHC gene products is not a general phenomenon and appears to be under epigenetic control which is not fully understood at present. More generally, regulation of HLA class II genes appears to be quite complex. We could not induce HLA-DR expression in T-lymphoma-derived cell lines upon -γ treatment. This result is in contradiction to the well-known inducibility of HLA class II expression on activated T lymphocytes from PHA or MLR stimulation. Such a contradiction might result from three different factors. Firstly, a molecule other than -γ may also be involved in HLA class II induction on PHA-stimulated lymphocytes. Indeed, we could not block the induction of HLA class II molecules on PHA-stimulated peripheral T lymphocytes by means of monoclonal antibodies directed against -γ. In such a case, however, -γ alone should not be able to induce HLA-DR expression on isolated T lymphocytes. Secondly T-lymphoma-derived cell lines may not belong to the same cell type as peripheral T lymphocytes able to express HLA-DR upon -γ treatment. T-lymphoma-derived cell lines usually express T-cell-specific antigens corresponding to a certain pathway of differentiation. T-lymphoma-derived cell lines might be blocked in such a path way. Thirdly resting T cells do not express detectable levels of -γ receptor (such results have been suggested by M. Rubinstein, personal communication).

C Induction of Non-MHC Genes by IFN

IFN-γ has been shown to induce the expression of a 12K polypeptide in human U937 cells as well as in human mononuclear cells. This polypeptide has significant amino acid homology to platelet factor 4 and β-thromboglobulin, two chemostatic proteins released by platelets on degranulation (Luster *et al.*, 1985).

D Effect of IFN on Variant Cell Lines That Do Not Express MHC Antigens

As we proceed in this review, the idea clearly arises that IFN is a powerful tool in the understanding of MHC gene regulation. Conversely, MHC genes might allow us to design models for IFN action on eucaryotic genes. Several variant human cell lines are now available that fail to express either class I or class II MHC antigens. These variants were either obtained spontaneously or specially selected for this property (Table III).

We wondered whether IFN might be able to induce the expression of the abnormally silent MHC genes in these cell lines. We therefore treated these cells with IFN-α, -β or -γ and analysed the effect on MHC class I as well as class II proteins and/or corresponding mRNAs. Except for the case of K562 described above, IFN could not induce expression of MHC genes that were abnormally silent in these variants.

TABLE III Human Lymphoblastoid cell lines variants MHC Expression

Name	Cell type	Expected expression	Expression in the variants	Spontaneous or selected *in vitro*
K562	Erythroleukemia Precursor?	?	–	Spontaneous
DAUDI	Burkitt lymphoma (B-cell line)	Class I and II	Class II only	id
T51-616	B-cell line	Class I and II	Class I only	Selected
Raji-Acola	id	id	id	id
T21-AoBo	id	id	Class II only	Selected
721-84,5	id	id	Class I only	id

Class I: Human lymphoblastoid cell line (HLCL) variants

DAUDI: This cell line does not synthesize or express β2m. This protein is now known to be necessary for the expression of HLA class I antigens. Quite surprisingly, DAUDI cytoplasm contains a β2m mRNA, as detected by hybridization (Rosa *et al.*, 1983b). Further studies have shown that this mRNA is not functional because its initiation codon has been mutated from ATG (methionine) to ATC (leucine). However, both HLA heavy-chain class I mRNA and β2m mRNA levels are increased upon IFN treatment. Therefore, the IFN effect on MHC antigens expression does not need the antigens to be normally expressed on the cell surface.

721-AoBo: No IFN treatment could induce class I MHC expression in this cell line, while β2m is normally synthesized. This finding is in good agreement with the set of evidence that "classical" HLA-A, B genes have been deleted in this cell upon mutagenesis and selection (Orr and De Mars, 1983).

Class II: Human lymphoblastoid cell line variants

721-84, 5: Neither type I IFN nor IFN-γ treatment could induce the synthesis of HLA-DR antigens in this cell line. This finding is in agreement with the reported deletion of the corresponding genes (Auffray *et al.*, 1983).

T51-616: The case of this variant is particularly interesting. T51-616 has been obtained from the human EBV-transformed B cell line T51 by immunoselection against HLA-DR antigens. This cell line does not express *any* of the class II MHC antigens or mRNA. Therefore HLA-DR, DQ and DP genes appear to be coordinately regulated (Levine *et al.*, 1985). Further studies have led these authors to the hypothesis that the normal B cell line contains a

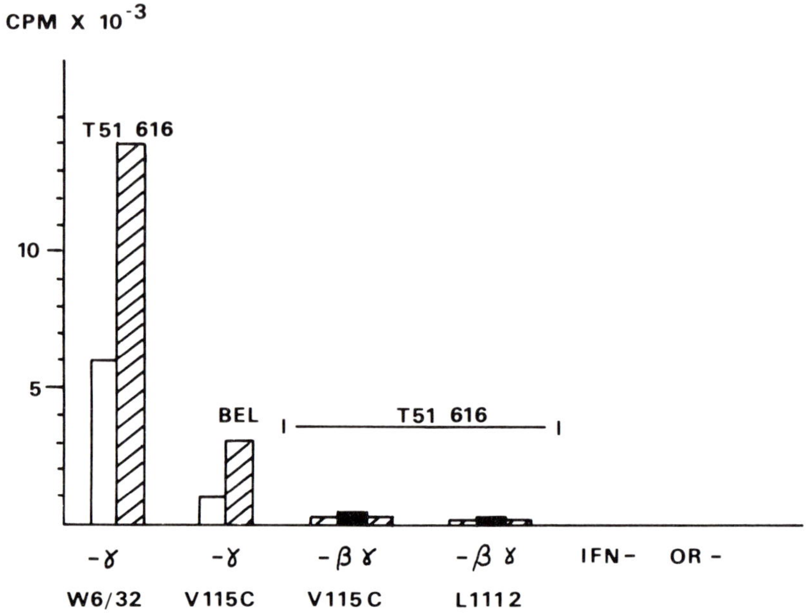

Fig. 6 Effect of IFN-γ on class II cell surface antigens in T51-616. T51, T51-616 or BEL cells were treated for 24 hours with IFN-β (hatched) or IFN-γ (solid) and HLA class I (W6/32) or HLA class II (V115C, L11, 12) cell surface antigens were measured by cellular radioimmunoassay (Rosa *et al.*, 1983c).

trans-acting element that positively regulates class II expression. For some reason, this activator is no longer active in the T51-616 cell line. We reasoned that IFN-γ might generally regulate HLA class II expression through the activation of this positive trans-acting element. Therefore, IFN-γ could be able to restore class II MHC expression in T51-616. However, neither IFN-α, -β nor IFN-γ could induce the expression of MHC class II HLA-DR antigens (Fig. 6). This suggests that either the positive trans-acting element required for class II expression in B cells is irreversibly inactive (by deletion of the corresponding gene, for instance) or that IFN-γ regulates HLA class II gene expression through a pathway that does not involve the class II activator. Similar conclusions were drawn from the study of another class II variant cell line (Long *et al.*, 1984).

E Conclusion

IFN appears to be both a modulator, able to increase the level of a MHC gene product already synthesized and expressed, and a real inducer, able to induce the "*de novo*" activation of at least two classes of MHC genes. One could argue that "regulation" usually means you can either "decrease" or "increase" the level of the gene expression studied. Up to now, IFN has been shown only to increase MHC gene expression. In some instances however, we repeatedly observed that instead of increasing class I MHC expression on mouse LM fibroblast cells for instance, IFN-treatment decreased the number of class I molecules at their surface. The basis for such an unexpected finding remains unknown. IFN could exert a particular negative effect on the cell membrane that would interfere with the enhancement of MHC expression derived from the enhancement of the corresponding mRNAs. In particular, such an effect of IFN on the cell membrane could explain why enhancement of the cell surface antigen by IFN is always lower than enhancement of the corresponding mRNA (Rosa *et al.*, 1983a). More generally, it is conceivable that, depending on the cell type studied, IFN might increase *or* decrease the level of MHC gene products in this cell line. Whatever its mechanism, MHC gene regulation by IFN suggests a role of major biological importance for IFN which is not restricted to its antiviral activity.

Our experiments on K562 (Sutherland *et al.*, 1985) and reports on the effects of IFN-γ on the expression of MHC class II antigens suggest that IFN might be involved in the differentiation of particular systems and may even be considered as a differentiation factor. In particular, the ability of IFN-γ to strongly enhance class II antigen expression on macrophages may augment the capacity of these cells to perform antigen presentation, which is Ia restricted. We shall discuss this result in Section V. However, the ability of IFN-γ to promote the appearance of MHC class II antigens on cells which do not spontaneously express them, such as skin fibroblasts and endothelial cells, may suggest an involvement of this lymphokine in the generation of autoimmune disease such as those described by Klareskog *et al.* (1982), and, more generally, an involvement of this type of cell in immune processes.

Is IFN a new class of inducer?

The ability of IFN to induce the expression of several genes increases the degree of similarity of this molecule to a hormone. We have compared the characteristic properties of different types of gene inducers, among which are hormones (Table IV).

Thus IFN has many characteristics in common with hormones, particularly IFN-γ. However, three main differences exist that render IFN an original cell effector. Firstly, IFN is the general name of a biological activity shared by three classes of molecules, which have common properties (antiviral activity, MHC class I regulation) and distinct properties (regulation of MHC class II genes, regulation of 2.5A synthetase). Secondly, IFN, when regulating class I genes, does not act on a specific differentiated

TABLE IV Comparison of Various Gene Inducers

	Heat-shock	Hormone	Lymphokine	IFN
Specificity of target tissue	No	Yes	Yes	Yes class II and No class I
Production by specific tissue	No	Yes	Yes	Yes Type II and No Type I
Circulates through blood stream	No	Yes	Acts locally?	Yes
Acts through a specific receptor	No	Yes	Yes	Yes
May act on a gene family	Yes	Yes	?	Yes
Biological nature	Physical parameter	Steroid or protein or else (?)	Protein or else (?)	Proteins

cell. However, IFN-γ regulates MHC class II gene expression in a restricted number of cell types. Thirdly, type I IFN is not produced by a specific tissue, whereas IFN-γ is. Therefore, IFN-γ appears to correspond more to a hormone than type I IFN.

III MECHANISM OF IFN ACTION ON MHC GENES

In eukaryotic cells, RNA accumulation is the result of three consecutive phenomena: transcription of the corresponding gene: processing of the primary nuclear transcript (Darnell, 1982) that goes along with the transfer of RNA into the cytoplasm; and RNA turnover inside the cell. Therefore, the modification of the cytoplasmic concentration of a specific RNA as well as the induction of its accumulation into the cytoplasm can be obtained through modifications of transcription, processing or degradation of this RNA. In most cases studied, induction of specific mRNA is due to an increased transcription of the corresponding gene (IFN, prolactin, growth hormone) (Raj and Pitha, 1983; Evans *et al.*, 1982). In some instances the induction of specific mRNA is obtained through an increased stability of this mRNA in the cytoplasm (casein, ovalbumin) (Darnell, 1982).

We reasoned that, since IFN was able to induce the expression of silent MHC genes in K562 or skin fibroblasts, it should most probably act at the level of transcription. We therefore studied the effect of IFN on the transcription rates of β2m, HLA class I and HLA class II genes.

Quantification of the rate of transcription of a specific gene is usually carried out by incorporation of a radiolabelled precursor into primary transcript. For abundant mRNA, incorporation of the labelled precursor is done on whole living cells (Darnell, 1982) with tritiated uridine. However, in that case, cells must be pulse-labelled (less than 10 minutes) to avoid secondary phenomena (stabilization). Furthermore, since the specific activity of tritiated uridine is quite low, incorporation of this isotope does not suit transcription rate measurement of genes with low activity. The recent availability of an *in vitro* transcription method using the so-called "isolated nuclei" (nuclear "run off") has allowed us to overcome these problems (Weber *et al.*, 1979).

RNA polymerases from "isolated nuclei" are able to carry out elongation of the nascent RNA chain. However, they cannot promote the initiation of new RNA molecules. Thus incorporation of radiolabelled nucleotides in RNA allows one to quantify the number of RNA polymerase per gene at the very time when nuclei were isolated from cells. One can therefore estimate the rate of transcription initiation of specific genes as a function of external conditions applied to the cell (Weber *et al.*, 1977).

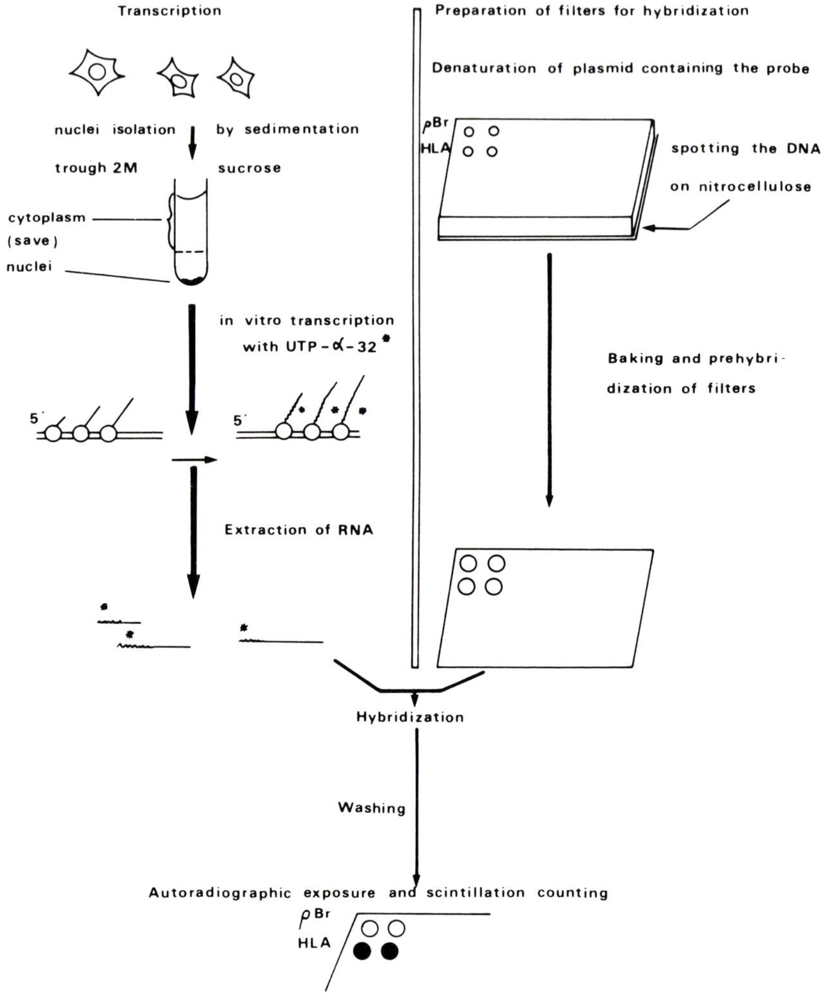

Fig. 7 Method of preparation of nuclei, and DNA-bound filter to study transcription rates.

A Effect of INF-β and IFN-γ on β2m and HLA-A, B, C Transcription Rates

We have used the method of isolated nuclei in order to quantify the transcription rate of HLA-A, B, C and β2m genes in the human BEL melanoma cell line. Following treatment of cells with IFN-β or -γ at 500 U/ml, nuclei were isolated according to Fig. 7 and incubated with ^{32}P-UTP (Schibler *et al.*, 1983). RNA has then been extracted and hybridized to

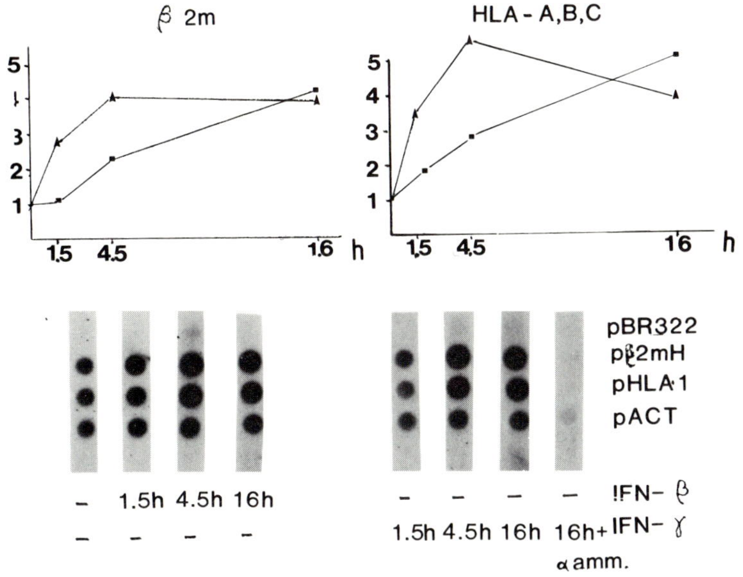

Fig. 8 Effect of IFN-β on HLA class I and β2m genes transcription. BEL cells were treated for various times with 500 U/ml IFN-γ or -β. Nuclei were isolated and run-off assay was performed. Newly synthesized RNA were isolated and hybridized to an excess of filter-bound DNA corresponding to β2m or HLA class I cDNA. Filters were then washed and exposed to XAR-5 films. Radioactivity was measured by densitometric scanning of the autoradiogram. *Lower part*: autoradiogram of filters. *Upper part*: kinetic of transcription rates stimulation of HLA. Class I and β2m genes: the relative increase in transcription rate is represented as a function of the incubation time of cells with IFN-γ (■) and IFN-β (▲).

an excess of filter-bound DNA from plasmids pBR322, pβ2mH (containing a β2m cDNA insert), pHLA (HLA cDNA insert), pACT (actin cDNA insert). Filters were then washed and exposed to XAR-5 films. Radioactivity retained on each spot is estimated by densitometric scanning of the autoradiogram.

Incubation of BEL cells with IFN-β or -γ induces an increase in the transcription of β2m and HLA-A, B, C detectable after one hour. The enhancement of transcription continues and is maintained for at least 16 hours (5-fold increase) (Fig. 8). However, the kinetics of enhancement of β2m and HLA gene transcription rates are slower when cells are incubated with IFN-γ than with IFN-β.

Therefore, both IFN-β and INF-γ promote an enhancement of transcription rates of β2m and HLA genes. IFN-α, -β and -γ have also been shown by others selectively to increase transcription rates of several genes such as HLA-A, B, C (Friedman and Stark, 1985), *p56* (Larner *et al.*, 1984), an early response gene (Luster *et al.*, 1985).

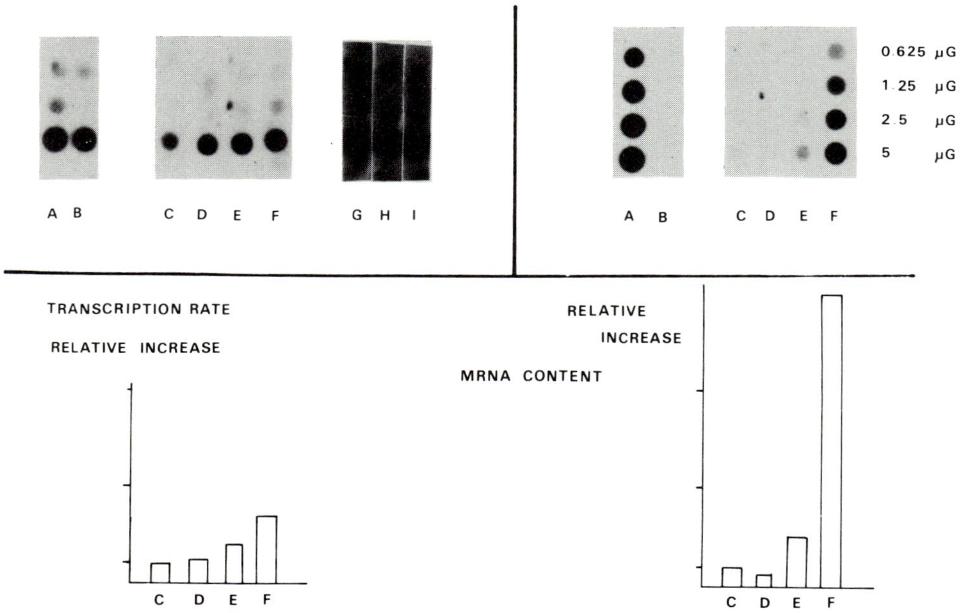

Fig. 9 Effect of IFN-β and IFN-γ on class II transcription and mRNA levels in VAL melanoma cell lines and JDA_2 fibroblast cell lines. VAL or JDA_2 cells were treated for 9 or 24 hours with IFN-β or -γ and analysed as in Fig. 8. Class II mRNA contents were measured by DOT-BLOT assay. Left: *Nuclear runoff assay*. On each filter, the order of cDNA DOTS is from top to bottom: β2m, HLA-DRα, HLA class I. Upper part: autoradiogram. Lower part: result of densitometric scanning. Right: *Class II mRNA levels measurements*. 5, 2.5, 1.25 or 0.625 μg of cytoplasmic mRNA were spotted on to nitrocellulose and hybridized to a class II cDNA probe (Rosa *et al.*, 1983a). Upper part: autoradiogram. Lower part: result of densitometric scanning.

A:	721 cells,	C, G:	no treatment
B:	721-84.5 cells	D, H:	IFN-β at 1000 U/ml for 24 hours
C, D, E, F:	VAL cells	E:	IFN-γ at 500 U/ml for 9 hours
G, H, I:	JDA_2 cells	F, I:	IFN-γ at 500 U/ml for 24 hours

B Effect of IFN on Class II Transcription

IFN-γ enhances the level of HLA class II mRNA and gene activity in melanomas. Moreover, IFN-γ induces the activity of silent class II genes in skin as well as endothelial fibroblasts. We therefore studied the effect of IFN-γ and -β on the transcription of HLA-DRα genes in two different cell lines VAL and JDA_2. VAL is a human melanoma cell line that expresses a high level of HLA class II mRNA. JDA_2 is an SV40-transformed skin fibroblast.

Treatment of VAL cells with IFN-γ at 500 U/ml for 24 hours slightly increases the transcription rate of HLA-DRα genes as shown in Fig. 9 (3-fold increase). Kinetic studies have shown that the increase in HLA-DRα transcription is slow (scarcely detectable after 4 hours). IFN-β had no effect on HLA-DRα transcription. In the same experiment, we measured the transcription rate of HLA-DRα gene in the human B lymphoblastoid cell line 721 and its DR-negative variant 721-84.5. No HLA-DRα transcription could be detected in the 721-84.5 cell line. The weak enhancement of HLA-DRα transcription in VAL cells upon IFN-γ treatment was in contrast to our previous results on the effect of IFN-γ on HLA-DRα mRNA levels in VAL cells. Indeed IFN-γ treatment for 24 hours at 500 U/ml strongly enhances HLA-DRα mRNA levels in VAL cells (15-20 fold) as demonstrated by dot-blot hybridization (Fig. 9). Therefore, the increase in transcription of HLA-DRα gene does not alone explain the strong increases of HLA-DRα levels in VAL cells.

We have also studied the effect of IFN-γ on HLA-DRα transcription in human JDA_2 skin fibroblasts by nuclear "run off" assay. There is no detectable HLA-DRα transcription in JDA_2 cells. IFN-γ (but not IFN-β) induces the transcription of HLA-DRα in these cells (Fig. 9).

IV MODEL OF IFN ACTION ON *MHC* GENE EXPRESSION

A DNA Target Sequence

What makes a gene specifically sensitive to IFN regulation?

Since IFNs transcriptionally regulate a discrete number of genes which are, at least in part, independent, one might assume that these genes share some common targets. Two types of factors might be involved in the specific control of one gene by one effector. The gene itself might carry specific sequences that are genetic targets for the effector. On the other hand, the environment of the gene itself might be involved in this control. Up until now, regulation of many genes, among them IFN, actin and albumin could be attributed to the presence of a specific DNA sequence, generally located within the gene itself or at the 5′ flanking region of its promoter. Such sequences have been located at −730 bp for rat heart actin (Melloul *et al.*, 1984), −720 bp for rat insulin (Walker *et al.*, 1983), −400 bp for rat albumin (Ott *et al.*, 1984).

We have tried to define whether the environment or the gene itself is involved in the specific regulation of an HLA class I gene by IFN. If a recombinant HLA gene is introduced by DNA transfection in a stable manner, in a murine cell, its environment may be modified since the integration of this HLA gene into the mouse genome is realized at random (Scangos and Ruddle, 1981). Therefore, products of the transfected genes will still be regulated by IFN if the HLA gene itself carries specific DNA sequences related to IFN sensitivity.

Complete HLA genes and IFN regulation. We could show that an HLA-A3 gene transfected into mouse L cells is regulated by mouse IFN, but is no longer induced by human IFN (Rosa *et al.*, 1983c). Indeed, mouse IFN, but not human IFN, treatment, increases the steady state level of HLA-A3 mRNA in transfected mouse L cells. We therefore postulated that IFN regulation of MHC class I genes can be divided at least into two steps. One step should be species-specific, since human IFN can no longer regulate a human gene in a murine cell line. The next step(s) should be non-species-specific since *mouse IFN* can regulate a *human* HLA gene. Species specificity in that case suggested that IFN acts on MHC class I genes through species-specific cell surface receptors for IFN.

The effect of IFN on MHC human class I genes transfected into mouse or Chinese hamster cells was also demonstrated by other laboratories (Gresser, 1983). Since a human HLA gene is regulated when it is transferred in another environment, the HLA gene in itself must carry specific sequences or a specific structure that is the genetic target for IFN action. The system of transfected genes provides a useful tool to study the genetic target for IFN action.

Truncated MHC class I genes and IFN regulation. If specific sequences for IFN sensitivity are present inside or around the HLA class I gene, one might expect that partial deletion of these sequences in HLA class I genes should abolish the sensitivity of this gene to IFN. This hypothesis could be studied through the combination of genetic engineering and DNA-mediated gene transfer. Yoishie *et al.* (1984) have generated HLA-B7 genes truncated at their 5′ end. They studied the effect of IFN on these truncated HLA genes when introduced into mouse L cells. Quite surprisingly, some HLA-B7 transfected clones of mouse L cells expressed the HLA-B7 specificity even if the promoter of the HLA-B7 gene had been deleted. These cells contain two types of HLA-B7 mRNA; one has the normal 1.8 Kb size, the other HLA-B7

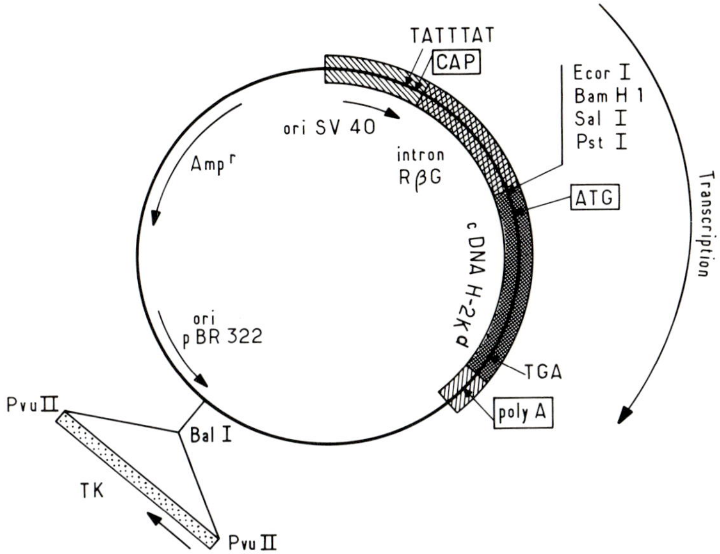

Fig. 10 Structure of plasmid pH-2^d SV33. TATTTAT: SV40 promoter. RBG: rabbit β-globin intron. ATG: initiation codon. TGA: termination codon. TK: thymidine kinase gene (from *Herpes simplex* virus). Poly A: SV40 polyadenylation sequence. CAP: transcription start.

mRNA is smaller than 1.8 Kb. Both HLA-B7 transcripts are stimulated by IFN treatment. The conclusion of Yoishie *et al.* is that the sequences for IFN sensitivity are located within HLA-B7 gene itself. Generation of HLA-B7 transcripts from HLA-B7 gene whose promoter has been deleted *in vitro*, could be explained either by the existence of a cryptic promoter inside the gene, or because the truncated HLA-B7 gene has recombined with the homologous MHC genes of LM cells, through gene transfer. Such a recombinational event was indeed described for MHC class I truncated genes (Goodenow *et al.*, 1983).

We tried to determine which part of MHC class I genes determines sensitivity to IFN. In particular, we wondered whether exons contain regulatory sequences. Using a full-length H-2K^d cDNA (Lalanne *et al.*, 1983), Cochet and Kourilsky have constructed a plasmid pH-2^d SV33 (Fig. 10) that allows the expression of the H-2K^d cDNA in eukaryotic cells. For this purpose, H-2K^d cDNA was introduced into pSVE vector (Harris and Breathnach, 1982) between the rabbit β globin intron and the SV40 early mRNA polyadenylation signal. In this construct, the transcription of the H-2K^d mRNA is under the control of the early promoter of SV40. We studied the effect of IFN on pH2^d SV33 expression when this plasmid is stably introduced into mouse L cells. As shown in Fig. 11, IFN could not stimulate H-2K^d mRNA levels in cells transfected with pH2^d SV33. Thus H-2K^d cDNA does not carry all sequences (if any) sensitive to IFN.

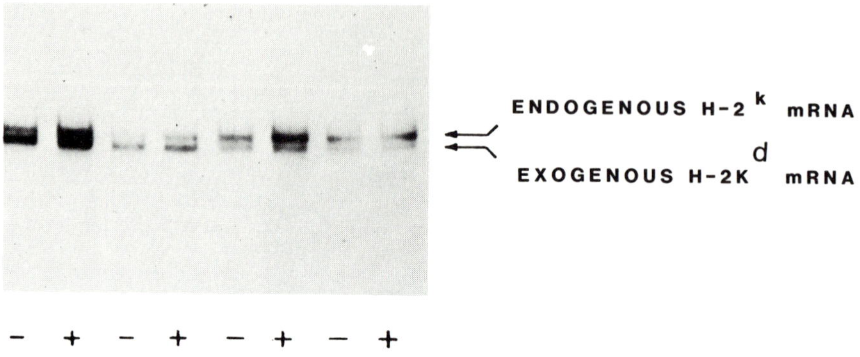

Fig. 11 Effect of IFN type I on H-2 mRNA levels in L cells transfected with pH-2^{d} SV 33. Four independent clones of L cells transfected with pH-2^{d} SV 33 were treated (+) or not treated (−) with murine IFN (type I). mRNA were extracted, resolved on an agarose–methylmercury hydroxide gel, transferred to nitrocellulose and hybridized to an H-2 cDNA probe (Lalanne *et al.*, 1983). Filters were washed and exposed to XAR-5 films. The upper band is derived from endogenous H-2 genes. The lower band, which is not found in parental L cells mRNA is derived from plasmid pH-2^{d} SV 33.

Consensus DNA sequences in genes regulated by interferons. IFN-α stimulates the transcription of several genes. Friedman and Stark (1985) postulated that such a coordinated transcriptional regulation could be due to the presence of a common regulatory sequence shared by all IFN-α-regulated genes. They compared the sequences of four human genes that are sensitive to IFN regulation: 2 HLA class I genes, 1 metallothionein gene, 1 HLA-DRα gene. They defined a consensus sequence, 30 nucleotides long:

$$\mathrm{TTCN}^{\mathrm{G}}_{\mathrm{C}}\mathrm{NACCTCNGCAGTTTCTC}^{\mathrm{C}}_{\mathrm{T}}\mathrm{TCT\text{–}CT}$$

This sequence is located in the 5′ flanking sequences of the four genes studied. However, its position varies from −145 from the transcription start (class I) to ∼ −600 (class II). Up until now, this sequence has been established only from a comparison of sequences. The role of this consensus sequence in IFN-directed regulation of genes could be demonstrated by using at least two different approaches.

Firstly one could either delete or mutate this sequence in the corresponding genes and study the effect of IFN on these modified genes. Secondly studies could be carried out on recombinant hybrid genes composed of this sequence ligated to a non-IFN-regulated gene such as the bacterial chloramphenicol acetyltransferase (CAT) gene. Such hybrid constructions between a H-2K^{d} promoter and the CAT gene have been constructed by Israel and Kourilsky and were recently shown to be sensitive to IFN action in preliminary experiments (A. Israel, personal communication).

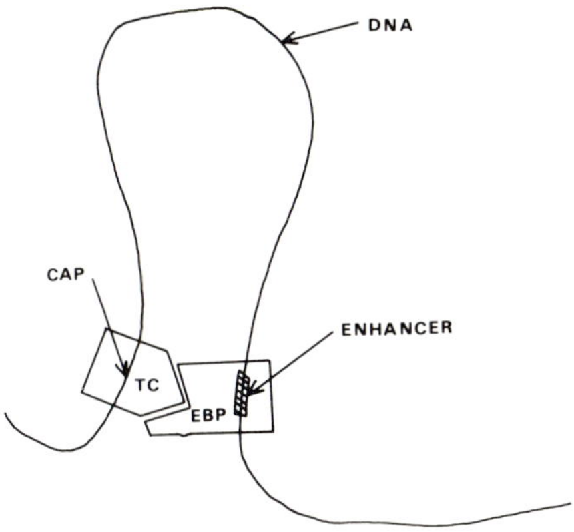

Fig. 12 Model for enhancer action. CAP: transcription start. EBP: enhancer binding protein. TC: transcription complex.

Is this consensus sequence an "enhancer"?

Enhancer sequences are cis-acting elements, different from promoters, with a characteristic structure (inverted repeats) that controls the level of transcription of specific genes (viral transcription, for instance) and confers tissue specificity to the expression of several genes (immunoglobulin or globin) (Dynan and Tjian, 1985). Enhancer elements can act at a great distance from the promoter, and their activity is not dependent upon their orientation. The consensus sequence described by Friedman and Stark (1985) could behave like an "enhancer". However, its structure is not characteristic of enhancer structure. Secondly, studies performed by Kimura have shown that an enhancer is present in H-2 class I genes close to the consensus sequence but different from it (Kimura *et al.*, 1986). Therefore, the IFN regulation consensus sequence is probably clearly different from a classical enhancer. However, it remains possible that it shares some properties with enhancers. Enhancers are now known to interact with DNA binding proteins; it has been proposed (Chambon, 1984) that enhancers can act at distance from a promoter (1–2 kb) according to the scheme of Fig. 12. Rather than opening DNA immediately close to the enhancer sequences, enhancer binding protein (EBP) would recognize another DNA binding protein such as specific transcription initiation factor (or RNA polymerase II) and activate it or induce its activity.*

*We recently demonstrated that both ICS and enhancer DNA sequences present in H-2 class I promoter are necessary for IFN-α, -β and -γ regulation. (A. Israel personal communication.)

IFN sensitivity could be mediated through the consensus sequence (ICS) described by Friedman. In particular, ICS could bind to a specific protein that would directly or indirectly activate the transcription of the neighbouring genes. Thus it would be of interest to demonstrate whether specific proteins are able to bind to ICS. This could be done by footprint analysis (incubating ICS with a whole-cell extract or nuclear extract from cells treated with IFN) (Dynam and Tjian, 1985). On the other hand, one could introduce by transfection a large amount of ICS in a cell and show (dilution analysis) that this can prevent the control of class I transcription by IFN.

How can we explain IFN-γ specificity toward class II genes?

IFN-β cannot regulate class II transcription either in melanoma or fibroblast cell lines, whereas IFN-γ does. Therefore, a unique interferon consensus sequence cannot explain such a specificity. In fact the HLA-DR interferon consensus sequence is not identical to HLA class I ICS. Subtle differences in sequence might be responsible for an IFN-γ specific effect on class II genes. A DNA binding protein under the control of IFN-γ might have a high affinity for both class I and class II ICS, whereas DNA binding protein under the control of type I IFN would recognize only class I ICS. On the other hand a differential effect of IFN-γ on class II genes could be explained by a particular localization of the interferon consensus sequence in these genes.

However, the interferon consensus sequence does not explain all the effects of IFN on MHC regulation. In particular ICS cannot explain the clear post-transcriptional effect of IFN-γ on class II mRNA steady state level we recently observed (Section III).

B Model of IFN Action on MHC Genes

Little is known about the first step by which IFN acts on MHC genes or other genes. As a hormone, IFN first binds to a specific receptor (Aguet, 1980). IFN-α and -β interact with the same receptor whose gene has been located on human chromosome 21 (Revel *et al.*, 1976). IFN-γ does not interact with this IFN type I receptor (Branca and Baglioni, 1981).

IFN receptors are located in the cell membrane but no precise data concerning structure or activity are known yet. In particular, there are no data concerning all the processes that happen between IFN binding to its specific receptor and activation of several sets of genes, among which are MHC genes. Our knowledge about IFN mechanism of action is summarized in Fig. 13. Many protein hormones, when binding to their cell surface receptor, promote the production of a "second messenger", for instance cyclic AMP, that mediates hormone action. IFN binding could promote the

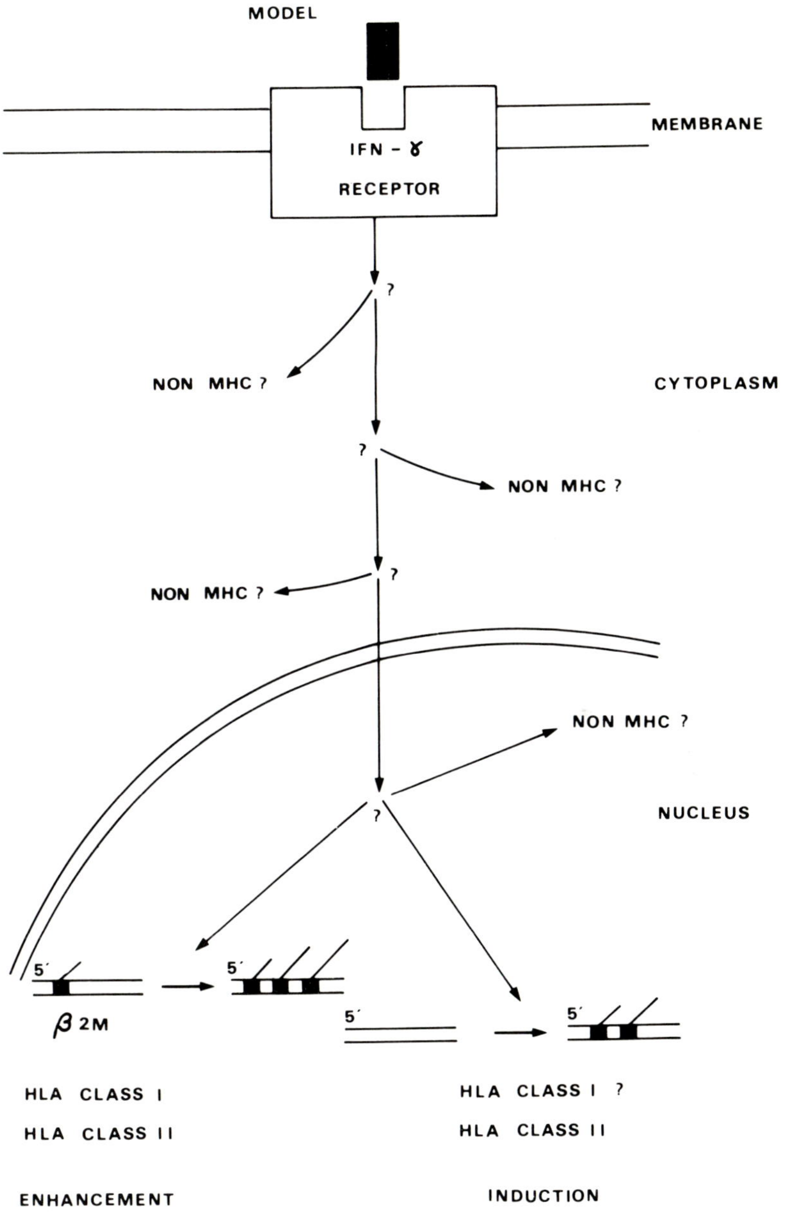

Fig. 13 Model for IFN biological activity.

production of such a second messenger. This messenger could activate several "proteins" or genes which would be involved in IFN biological activity. One way to demonstrate the existence of such "intermediate" genes or proteins would be to select a variant cell line resistant to certain effects of IFN. The effect of IFN on growth inhibition has been used to derive cell lines resistant to IFN (Lindahl *et al.*, 1973). However, growth inhibition upon IFN treatment might result from a complex phenomenon, not yet well known. On the other hand, IFN-directed MHC gene product activation appears to be a quite convenient tool to generate IFN-resistant cell lines.

V CONSEQUENCES OF IFN EFFECT ON MHC

A Genetic

In an attempt to understand better the mechanism of action of IFN on MHC genes, we studied the effect of human IFN-α, -β and -γ on the man–mouse–hybrid cell line WAVR4. This hybrid, whose human chromosome content is restricted to chromosome 21, has been shown to express human

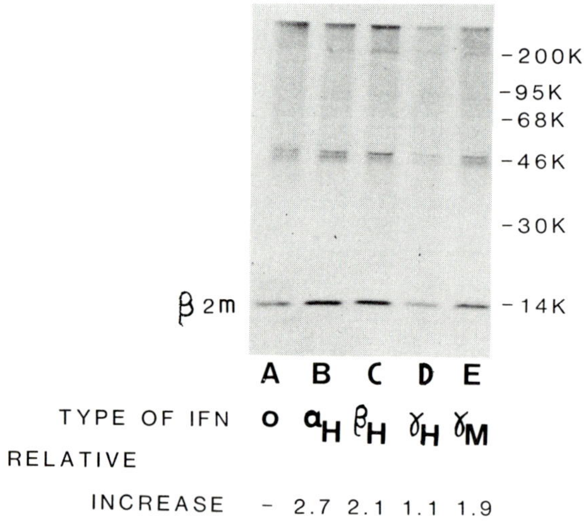

Fig. 14 Effect of human IFNs on β2m synthesis in WAVR4 cells. Following an overnight incubation with human IFN-α, -β, -γ or murine IFN-γ at 500 U/ml, WAVR4 cells were pulse-labelled, lysed and immunoprecipitated as described in Fig. 1, except that rabbit anti-mouse β2m was used as an immune serum instead of B 9.12.1 monoclonal antibody. A: no treatment. B: human IFN-α. C: human IFN-β. D: human IFN-γ. E: murine IFN-γ. Relative increase of β2m synthesis following IFN treatment was quantified by densitometric scanning of the autoradiograph and is represented under the picture. Reprinted from the *Annales de l'Institut Pasteur*, with permission.

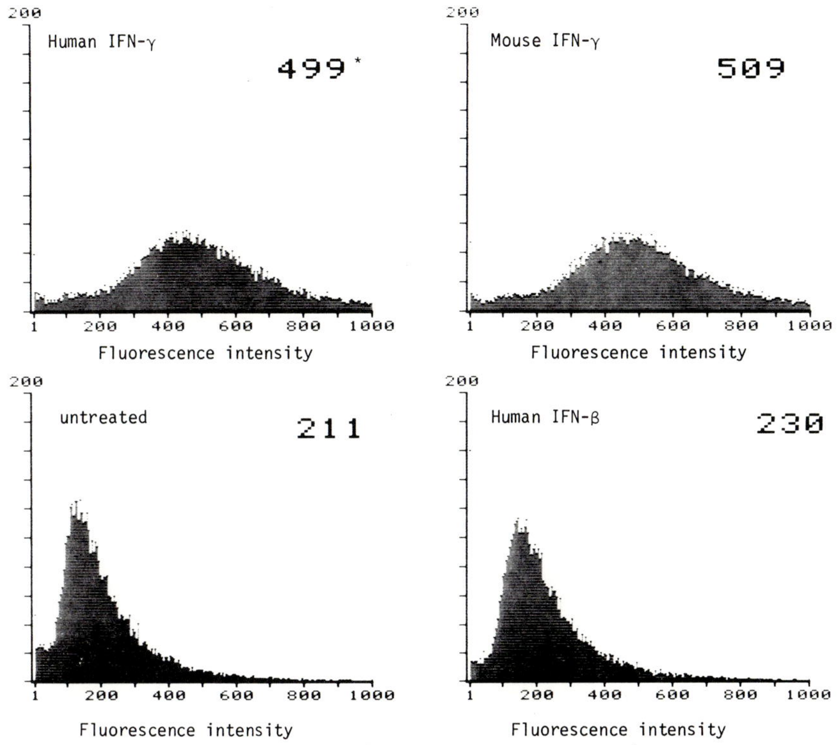

Fig. 15 Analysis of a somatic cell hybrid responding to human IFN-γ but not human IFN-β. Cells of this hybrid were treated with either human or murine IFN (as indicated) for 24 hours and analysed by quantitative immunofluorescence with anti-H-2^d monoclonal antibody.

IFN-α and -β receptors (Revel *et al.*, 1976). We confirm these results, since β2m protein synthesis in WAVR4 is enhanced upon human IFN-α or -β treatment (Fig. 14). As expected, human IFN-γ failed to enhance mouse β2m protein synthesis in WAVR4. Indeed, the gene for the IFN-γ receptor has been reported not to be located on chromosome 21 in man.

We have used the effect of IFN on H-2 class I antigens to localize genetically human IFN-γ receptor. Twenty-two independent man–mouse hybrids were tested for the coordinate segregation of human IFN-γ receptor (through its biological activity), a specific human chromosome and chromosome-specific enzyme marker (Fellous *et al.*, 1985). Man–mouse hybrids were labelled with a monoclonal anti-H-2 serum, revealed by fluorescein isothiocyanate-labelled IgG fraction of goat anti-mouse Ig (FITC-GAM). Results were analysed and quantified on a cytofluorometer. Figure 15 shows an example of one hybrid that responds to human IFN-γ but not -β by expressing

HUMAN IFN γ RECEPTOR/CHROMOSOME

Chromosome	+/+	-/-	+/-	-/+
1	5	8	3	4
2	3	8	5	4
3	6	5	2	7
4	4	6	4	6
5	3	6	5	6
6	6	6	2	6
7	4	3	4	9
8	6	5	2	7
9	0	11	8	1
10	4	9	4	3
11	5	5	2	7
12	6	2	2	10
13	1	9	7	3
14	1	9	7	3
15	2	9	6	3
16	4	8	4	4
17	5	1	3	11
18	8	12	0	0
19	6	5	2	7
20	6	3	2	9
21	5	3	3	9
22	3	6	5	6
X	1	6	7	6

Fig. 16 Coordinate segregation of human IFN-γ receptor and chromosome 18 in man/mouse hybrids.

more H-2 cell surface antigens following IFN-γ treatment. The analysis of segregation has shown (Fig. 16) that only hybrids carrying human chromosome 18 are sensitive to human IFN-γ. All other human chromosomes showed discordant segregation, including chromosome 21.

We are presently using the effect of IFN on MHC antigens to clone human IFN receptors according to the following scheme (in collaboration with M. Revel). Mouse cell line LM^{tk-} is sensitive to mouse IFN-β but not to human IFN-β (effect on H-2 class I antigens). The IFN-directed increase of H-2 class I antigens can be analysed by cytofluorography. Cell sorting can be used to isolate cells that respond to mouse IFN. Mouse LM^{tk-} cells have been transfected with human DNA and *Herpes simplex* virus Tk gene. Transfectants have been treated with human IFN-β. Cell sorting has been used to isolate transfectants that became sensitive to human IFN-β

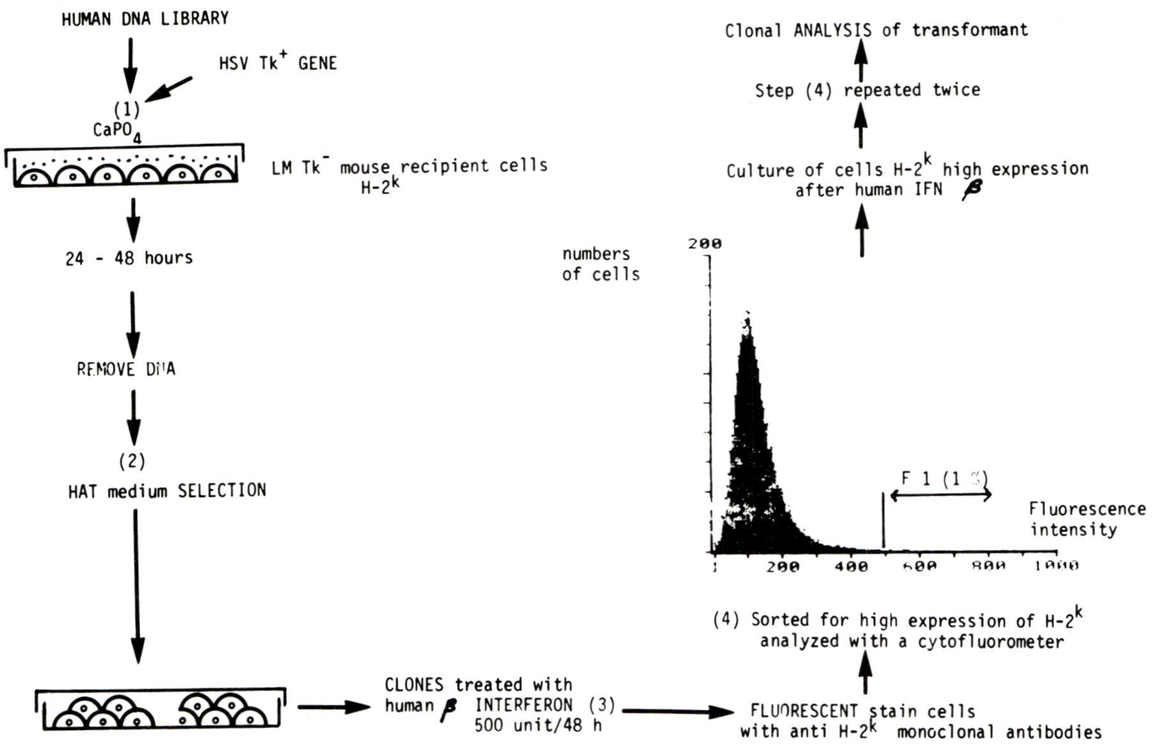

Fig. 17 Principle of human interferon receptors cloning (see text).

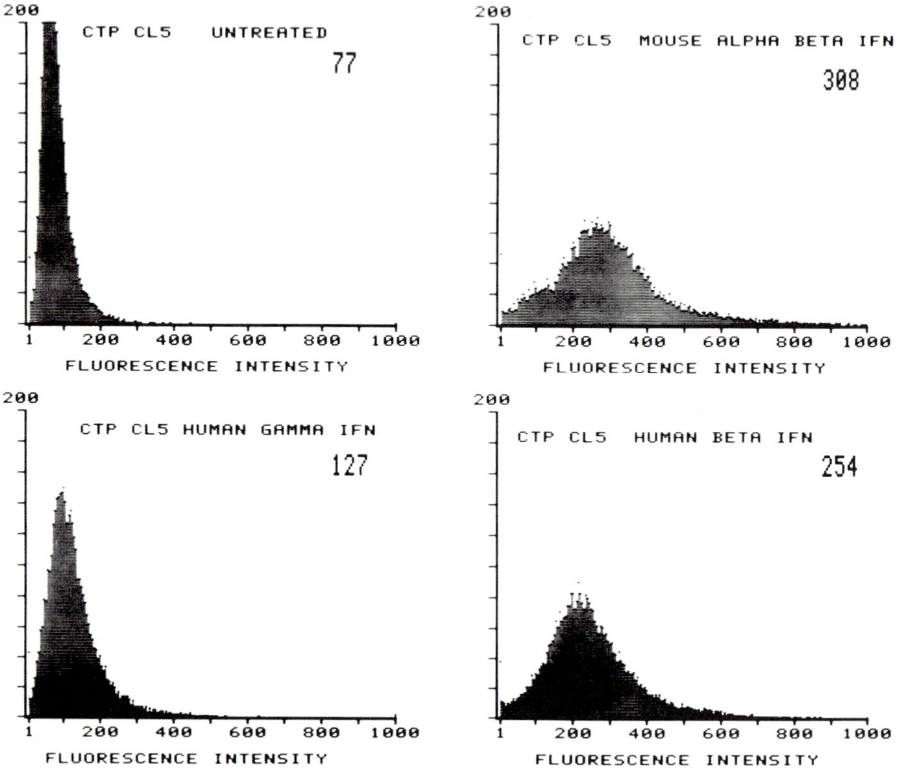

Fig. 18 Analysis of mouse LM cells transformant for the receptor of human interferon β. Cells were analysed as described in Fig. 15 (in colloboration with M. Revel).

(Fig. 17) (high expression of H-2 class I antigens following human IFN treatment. After several cycles of sorting, clones of transfected cells stably sensitive to human IFN-β were isolated (Fig. 18). We are presently isolating human genes present in those clones through human specific sequences (*Alu* sequence).

B Biological Significance of IFN-directed MHC Regulation

Is there any biological significance to the effect of IFN on MHC antigens?

Such a complex mechanism—allowing three different molecules to regulate a gene family involved in general immune survey—should play a physiological role. In particular, IFN-γ appears to be an excellent candidate for involvement in the physiological regulation of MHC class I and class II genes. We have attempted to study several models of *in vitro* immune reaction.

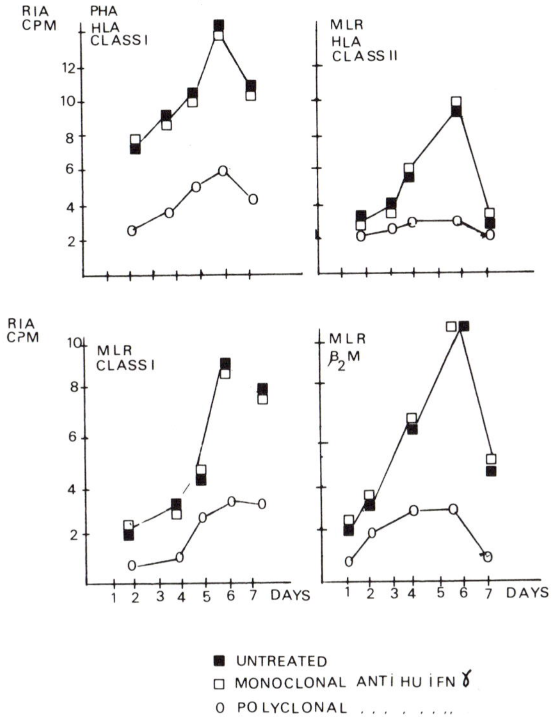

Fig. 19 Effects of anti human IFN-γ antibodies on HLA class I or class II antigen increase during MLR or PHA lymphocyte stimulation. MLR or PHA-stimulation was induced on peripheral blood lymphocytes. Every day, a cell aliquot was removed and cell surface antigen levels were measured as described in Fig. 6. Solid squares: control. Open squares: stimulation was performed in the presence of monoclonal antibodies anti-IFN-γ. Open circles: stimulation was performed in the presence of polyclonal antibodies anti-IFN-γ.

Mixed lymphocyte reaction (MLR) (collaborative work with E. Wollman, Institute Gustav Roussy, Villejuif). During MLR proliferative response, the amount of cell surface class I and class II antigens increases to peak at the sixth day of the reaction (Wollman and Kalil, 1983) (Fig. 19). -γ, produced in large amounts during MLR, could be responsible for such an increase. We have attempted to block such an increase by adding either polyclonal or monoclonal anti-IFN-γ antibodies at the beginning of the MLR process. Whereas polyclonal antibodies directed against IFN-γ prevent the increase of cell surface class I and class II antigens, monoclonal anti-IFN-γ antibodies could not block cell surface MHC antigen enhancement (Fig. 19). Therefore, if IFN-γ is partly involved in the enhancement of MHC antigens during MLR, its presence cannot alone control such events.

Such contradictory results might derive from several reasons:

(1) IFN-γ preparations are frequently contaminated by other lymphokines produced during MLR (Trinchieri and Perussia, 1985). Polyclonal antibodies anti-IFN-γ could recognize some of these lymphokines, involved in the enhancement of MHC antigens while monoclonal anti-IFN-γ antibodies could not. Indeed $BCGF_1$ has been reported to increase class II antigens on resting B lymphocytes.
(2) IFN-γ could act without being excreted into the culture medium. However, in such a case, polyclonal anti-IFN-γ antibodies could not block MHC antigen enhancement during MLR.

Effect of IFN-γ on antigen presentation. Antigen presentation is one of the first steps in the pathway of antibody production. T "helper" lymphocytes specifically recognize one antigen but require the help of macrophages. Macrophages are thought to trap the antigen, degrade it and "present" it in the MHC environment to T helper lymphocytes. When T helper lymphocytes specific for the antigen are mixed with the antigen and macrophages, they proliferate (Grey and Chesnut, 1985). Antigen presentation is restricted to class II MHC antigens. The efficiency of antigen presentation is proportional to class II MHC antigen concentration (Matis *et al.*, 1983).

We postulated that macrophages treated with IFN-γ (therefore expressing more MHC class II antigens) could present the antigen to T helper lymphocytes more efficiently. We thus studied (in collaboration with Dr J. J. Ballet, Hôpital St-Louis, Paris) the effect of IFN-γ on the efficiency of tetanus toxoid presentation by human macrophages (Fig. 20). The increase in antigen presentation efficiency is low (less than 60%). Similar results were obtained in the laboratory of P. Debré (Hôpital La Pitié, Paris). In a different system, Folsom *et al.* (1984) studied the effect of IFN-γ on ovalbumin presentation by tumour macrophage cell line P388D1 transfected with I-E^b_β gene. This cell line can present ovalbumin to $E^d_\alpha E^b_\beta$ restricted T cell hybridoma. P388D1-I-E^b_β cell line has a poor efficiency of ovalbumin presentation. If P388D1-I-E^b_β cells are treated with conA supernatant (culture medium from activated T lymphocytes which contains IFN-γ), the efficiency of ovalbumin presentation is increased 60-fold.

Folsom's result is in apparent contradiction to our results concerning the effect of IFN-γ on antigen presentation efficiency. This could be explained if we assumed that a threshold value of class II antigen expression on macrophage cell surface exists. Above this threshold value, further increases in macrophage class II cell surface antigen would not increase the efficiency of antigen presentation. Conversely, other lymphokines, present in conA supernatant but not in recombinant IFN-γ preparations, could be involved in the increase of antigen presentation efficiency.

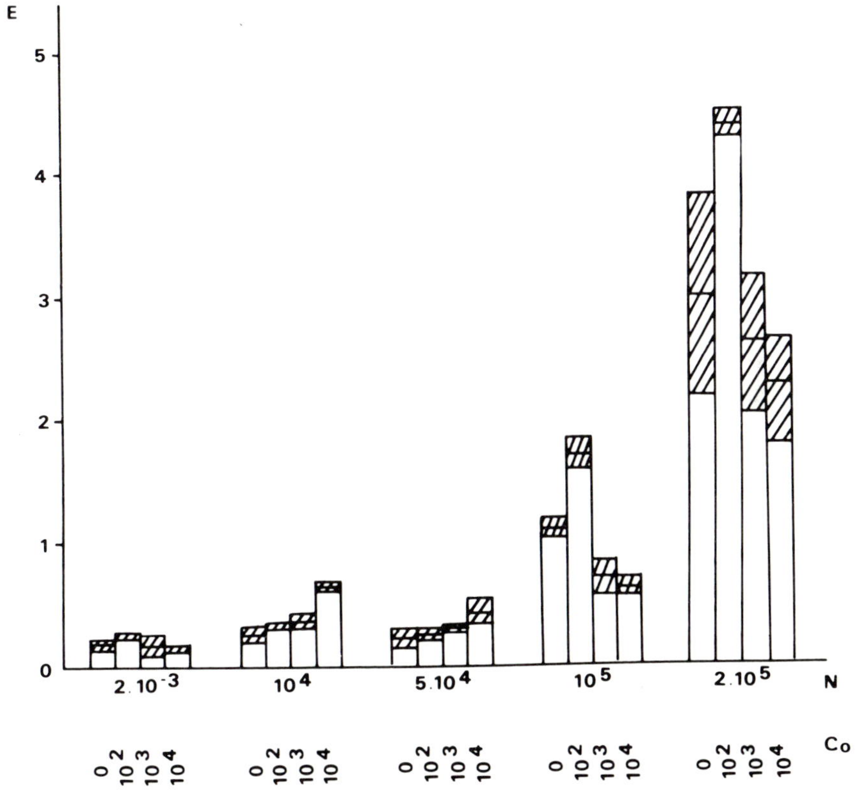

Fig. 20 Effect of IFN-γ on antigen presentation efficiency of human macrophages. Peripheral macrophages were treated for 24 hours with various concentration of IFN-γ (Co) and mixed with tetanus toxoid and cell from T cell clone specific for tetanus toxoid. T cell proliferation was measured by ^{3}H-thymidine incorporation. *N*: number of presenting macrophages/well. *E*: thymidine incorporation (c.p.m. $\times$ 10^{-3}).

Cytotoxic lysis by CTL. Cells infected by a virus often express a "viral" antigen at their surface. Cytotoxic lymphocytes (CTLs) specifically directed against the viral antigen are able to kill the cell that harbours this antigen. The recognition process is MHC class I or class II restricted; CTLs recognize and kill infected cells only if the infected cell carries MHC class I antigens that are identical to the MHC class I antigens carried by the effector CTLs. We postulated that the effect of IFNs on MHC antigen levels could be involved in the indirect elimination of viruses through CTL activity. That is, by increasing the number of MHC class I or class II molecules on cells treated, IFN could improve recognition of virus-infected cells by specific CTLs.

In an *in vitro* model system, we studied the efficiency of lysis by specific CTLs, directed against Influenza or Epstein-Barr virus antigens, of human cells infected with Influenza or Epstein-Barr viruses. Treatment of infected target cells by IFN did not lead to an increased sensitivity of these cell lines to CTL lysis (collaborative work with E. Gomard, Hôpital Cochin, Paris).

Shimonkevitz *et al.* (1985) have performed similar experiments. They have generated CTL clones directed against H-2K^d specificity. They studied the effect of IFN-γ treatment of target H-2K^d cells on their susceptibility to lysis by different clones of anti-H-2K^d CTLs. It is of interest that two types of anti-H-2K^d clones could be defined. For type A clones, IFN-γ treatment of target cells did not lead to an increased sensitivity of target cells to CTL lysis. For type B CTL clones, IFN-γ treatment dramatically increased susceptibility of target cells to lysis by the corresponding CTL clones. The data Shimonkevitz *et al.* presented "indicated a correlation between the differential ability of CTL clones to recognize and lyse target cells bearing minimal or optimal surface antigen (MHC) with their susceptibility to inhibition by anti-Lyt-2 antibody. In general, clones resistant to Lyt-2 inhibition (and hence bearing putative high-affinity antigen receptors) (Type A) were able to lyse target cells expressing low levels of antigen, whereas anti-Lyt-2 susceptible clones (bearing putative low-affinity antigen receptors) (Type B) could not. In two instances, this effect appeared to be just as dependent on the density of target cell allo-antigen (H-2K^d) as on CTL receptor affinity for antigen . . .". Therefore, IFN-γ may render IFN-γ-treated target cells sensitive to lysis by specific CTLs that carry low-affinity antigen receptor.

C Clinical Implications of IFN-directed MHC Regulation

Involvement of IFN-γ in autoimmunity

IFN-γ or conA treatment promotes the expression of class II antigens on cells that usually do not express these antigens. Unexpected expression of HLA class II antigens has been observed *in vivo* on different cell types: thyroid cells (Pujol-Borrel *et al.*, 1983; Londei *et al.*, 1984), endothelial fibroblast (Koyoama, 1979). IFN-γ could be responsible for this unexpected expression of HLA class II antigens on cells that usually do not express them. In such a case, these HLA class II positive cells may have the ability to present their own specific antigens to T helper lymphocytes. Such a process could generate immunity against auto-antigens from the cell type induced to abnormally express HLA class II antigens. Hence, IFN-γ could be involved in the generation of auto-immune diseases.

Bare lymphocyte syndrome

In some cases of immunodeficiencies, MHC antigens are not present at the cell surface of lymphocytes (bare lymphocyte syndrome).

MHC class I expression deficiency. Durandy *et al.* (1983) have investigated the inducibility of silent MHC class I genes by IFN in bare lymphocytes. They could induce *in vitro* cell surface expression of HLA class I antigens as well as β2m upon IFN-β treatment. Expression of HLA antigens by bare lymphocytes upon IFN treatment was demonstrated by microcomplement cytotoxicity assay using polymorphic antibodies as well as specific cytotoxic lysis by CTL. HLA specificities could be induced on PHA-stimulated bare lymphocytes after 24 hours' treatment with either IFN-α or IFN-β.

Two patients with class I deficiency have been treated with IFN-β (150,000 units per kg per day) for 7 days. This treatment lead to *in vivo* induction of HLA class I antigen expression as well as β2m expression. However, IFN treatment did not reduce immunodeficiency in these patients and did not prevent their death.

In recent studies, Grospierre and Virelizier (1986) reported similar experiments performed with IFN-γ. Interestingly, IFN-γ treatment could not induce either *in vitro* or *in vivo* expression of MHC class I antigens on bare lymphocytes.

MHC class II deficiency. In some cases of bare lymphocyte syndrome, B lymphocytes of patients do not express MHC class II antigens. In a recent meeting at Stanford University, B. Mach and collaborators reported the results of their studies on this type of deficiency (De Preval and Mach 1985). They have shown that no HLA class II mRNA is present in B bare lymphocytes. Genetic studies demonstrated that class II deficiency is probably due to the inactivation of a regulator gene, which segregates independently from chromosome 6. Interestingly, IFN-γ treatment could not induce the expression of class II genes in either B lymphocytes or skin fibroblasts from these patients. We fall then in a situation analoguous to variant class II negative human lymphoblastoid cell line T51–616 (described on p. 58).

VI GENERAL CONCLUSIONS

Our knowledge of IFN effects on MHC genes has been greatly increased by these new findings. However, several issues remain unanswered. Firstly, IFNs have been shown to interact with MHC class I and class II genes. It would be of interest to know whether regulation by IFN is a general property of

MHC genes (including class II) or is restricted to histocompatibility antigen genes (class I and class II). Secondly, it remains to be understood how a family of three classes of molecules with known antiviral activity (IFN), interacting with different receptors, can regulate a common set of genes (class I) or regulate different genes (class II). Such studies are underway in our laboratory. Thirdly, there remains the question that even though studies on the effect of IFN on MHC genes has led to a better knowledge of MHC genetic regulation, can we say that IFN *regulates* MHC expression?

Many experiments have been designed *in vitro* to prove that IFN are involved in immune regulation through their effect on MHC antigens. Of particular interest are those experiments suggesting that IFN-γ might help CTL with low-affinity antigen receptors to lyse target cells.

However there is no direct demonstration that *in vivo* IFN regulates MHC gene expression: that IFN is involved in physiological regulation—by decreasing or increasing MHC antigen levels—of MHC antigens. Furthermore, there is no *in vivo* direct data concerning the physiological significance of IFN effects on MHC genes. One way to demonstrate that IFN "regulation" of MHC genes is involved in immune regulation would be to construct *MHC* class I or class II genes with inactive IFN consensus sequence. Such mutated genes could be introduced into mouse eggs. One could study, using appropriate viruses or bacteria or antigens, the immune behaviour of such transgenic mice. But that is the future.

ACKNOWLEDGEMENTS

We thank Drs Malissen, Pious and Wiezerbin for the gifts of monoclonal antibodies B9.12.1, V1.15.C and recombinant IFN-γ. We thank Dr Rubinstein and Dr Novick for the gift of purified IFN-γ and -β. We thank Dr Revel for many helpful discussions and Dr E. Wollman for her help in performing the MLR inhibition assay. We thank Dr De Mars for variant cell lines 721, Dr Ballet and Dr Debré for performing the antigen presentation assays.

We thank Mrs M. Tassier for her help in typing the manuscript.

We would like to dedicate this work to Dr E. Fellous.

REFERENCES

Aguet, M. (1980). *Nature* (*London*) **284**, 459–460.

Auffray, C., Kuo, J., De Mars, R. and Strominger, J. L. (1983). *Nature* (*London*) **304**, 174–176.

Basham, T. Y. and Merigan, T. C. (1983). *J. Immunol.* **130**, 1492–1496.

Basham, T. Y., Bourgeade, M. F., Creasey, A. A. and Merigan, T. C. (1982). *Proc. Natl Acad. Sci. USA* **79**, 3265–3268.
Besançon, F. and Bourgeade, M. F. (1985). Colloque d'Animation INSERM, Génétique Moléculaire et Pathologie, Paris.
Branca, A. A. and Baglioni, R. (1981). *Nature (London)* **294**, 768–770.
Burrone, O. R. and Milstein, C. (1982). *EMBO J.* **1**, 345–349.
Chambon, P. (1984). Congress on Neoplastic cell and differentiation, Heidelberg.
Cochet & Kourilsky (unpublished results).
Darnell, J. E. Jr. (1982). *Nature (London)* **297**, 365–368.
De Preval, C. and Mach, B. (1985). IVth HLA and H-2 cloning meeting, Stanford.
Dolei, A. F., Ameglio, M. R., Capobianchi, T. and Tosi, R. (1981). *Antiviral Res* **1**, 367–373.
Durandy, A., Virelizier, J. L. and Grisielli, C. (1983). *Clin. Exp. Immunol.* **52**, 173–178.
Dynan, W. S. and Tjian, R. (1985). *Nature (London)* **316**, 774–776.
Esko, J. D., Gilmore, J. R. and Glaser, M. (1977). *Biochemistry* **16**, 1881–1890.
Evans, R. M., Birnberg, N. C. and Rosenfeld, M. G. (1982). *Proc. Natl Acad. Sci. USA* **79**, 7659.
Fellous, M., Kamoun, M., Gresser, I. and Bono, R. (1979). *Eur. J. Immunol.* **9**, 46–452.
Fellous, M., Nir, U., Wallach, D., Merlin, G., Rubinstein, M. and Revel, M. (1982a). *Proc. Natl Acad. Sci. USA* **79**, 3082–3086.
Fellous, M., Gunzburg, I. and Littauer, U. S. (1982b). *EMBO J.* **1**, 835–839.
Folsom, V., Gold, D. P., White, J., Marrack, P., Kappler, J. and Tonegawa, S. (1984). *Proc. Natl Acad. Sci. USA* **81**, 2045–2058.
Friedman, R. L. and Stark, G. R. (1985). *Nature (London)* **314**, 637–639.
Goodenow, R. S., Stroynowski, I., McMillan, M., Nicolson, M., Eakle, K., Taylor Sher, B., Davidson, N. and Hood, L. (1983). *Nature (London)* **301**, 388–392.
Grey, H. M. and Chesnut, R. (1985). *Immunology Today* **6**, 101–106.
Grospierre, J. and Virelizier, J. L. (1986). (in press).
Harris, B. A. and Breathnach, R. (1982). *Nucleic Acids Res.* **11**, 2615–2626.
Heron, I., Hokland, M. and Berg, K. (1978). *Proc. Natl Acad. Sci. USA* **77**, 6215–6219.
Hirsch, M. R., Wietzerbin, J., Pierres, M. and Goridis, C. (1983). *Neurosci. Lett.* **41**, 199–204.
Houghton, A. N., Thomson, T. M., Gross, D., Dettgen, H. F. and Old, L. J. (1984). *J. Exp. Med.* **160**, 255–269.
Jonak, J. and Knight, E. Jr. (1984). *Proc. Natl Acad. Sci. USA* **81**, 1747–1750.
Kimura, A., Israel, A., Le Bail, O. and Kourilsky, P. (1986). *Cell* **44**, 261–272.
Klareskog, L., Forsum, U., Scheynius, A., Kabelitz, D. and Wigzell, H. (1982). *Proc. Natl Acad. Sci. USA* **79**, 3632–3636.
Klein, E., Klein, G., Nadkarni, J. S., Wigzell, H. and Clifford, P. (1968). *Cancer Res.* **28**, 1300–1310.
Koeffler, H. P., Ranyard, J., Yelton, L., Billing, R. and Bohman, R. (1984). *Proc. Natl Acad. Sci. USA* **81**, 4080–4083.
Koyoama, Y. (1979). *Immunology* **38**, 383–390.
Lalanne, J. L., Delarbre, C., Gachelin, G. and Kourilsky, P. (1983). *Nucleic Acids Res.* **11**, 1567–1579.
Larner, C., Jonak, G., Creng, Y. S. E., Korant, B., Knight E. and Darnell, J. E. Jr. (1984). *Proc. Natl Acad. Sci. USA* **81**, 6733–6737.

Le Meur, M., Gerlinger, P., Benoist, C. and Mathis, D. (1985). *Nature* (*London*) **316**, 38–43.
Levine, F., Erlich, H. A., Mach, B. and Pious, D. (1985). *J. Immunol.* **134**, 1207–1213.
Lindahl, P., Leary, P. and Gresser, I. (1973). *Proc. Natl Acad. Sci. USA* **70**, 2785–2789.
Londei, M., Lamb, J. R., Bottazzo, G. and Feldmann, M. (1984). *Nature* (*London*) **312**, 639–641.
Long, E. D., Mach, B. and Accola, R. S. (1984). *Immunogenetics* **19**, 349–355.
Luster, A. D., Unkeless, J. C. and Ravetch, J. V. (1985). *Nature* (*London*) **315**, 672–676.
Matis, A., Glimcher, L. H., Paul, W. E. and Schwartz, R. H. (1983). *Proc. Natl Acad. Sci. USA* **79**, 6019–6023.
Melloul, D., Aloni, B., Calvo, J., Yaffe, D. and Nudel, O. (1984). *EMBO J.* **3**, 983–987.
Nakamura, M., Manser, T., Pearson, G. D. N., Daley, M. J. and Gefter, M. L. (1984). *Nature* (*London*) **307**, 381–382.
Orr, H. T. and De Mars, R. (1983). *Nature* (*London*) **302**, 534–536.
Ott, M. O., Sperling, L., Herbomel, P., Yaniv, M. and Weiss, M. C. (1984). *EMBO J.* **3**, 2505–2507.
Ploegh, H., Orr, M. T. and Strominger, J. L. (1981). *Cell* **24**, 287–293.
Pober, J. S., Gimbrone, M. A., Cotran, R. S., Reiss, C. S., Burakoff, S. J., Fiers, W. and Ault, K. A. (1983a). *J. Exp. Med.* **157**, 1339–1353.
Pober, J. S., Collins, T., Gimbrone, M. A. Jr., Cotran, R. S., Gitlin, J. D., Fiers, W., Clayberg, C., Kremsky, A. M., Burakoff, S. J. and Reiss, C. S. (1983b). *Nature* **305**, 726–729.
Potter, E., Nicolaisen, A. K., Ong, E. S., Evans, R. M. and Rosenfeld, M. G. (1981). *Proc. Natl Acad. Sci. USA* **78**, 6662–6666.
Pujol-Borrell, R., Hanafusa, T., Chiovato, L. and Bottazzo, G. F. (1983). *Nature* (*London*) **304**, 71–73.
Raj, B. K. and Pitha, P. M. (1983). *Proc. Natl Acad. Sci. USA* **80**, 3923–3927.
Revel, M., Bash D. and Ruddle, F. M. (1976). *Nature* (*London*) **260**, 139–143.
Rosa, F., Hatat, D., Abadie, A., Wallach, D., Revel, M. and Fellous, M. (1983a). *EMBO J.* **2**, 1585–1589.
Rosa, F., Berissi, H., Weissenbach, J., Maroteaux, L., Fellous, M. and Revel, M. (1983b). *EMBO J.* **2**, 239–243.
Rosa, F., Le Bouteiller, P. P., Abadie, A., Mishal, Z., Lemonnier, F. A., Bourrel, D., Lamotte, M., Kalil, J., Jordan, M. and Fellous, M. (1983c). *Eur. J. Immunol.* **13**, 495–499.
Rosa, F., Hatat, D., Abadie, A. and Fellous, M. (1985). *Ann. Immunol.* (*Inst. Pasteur*) **136C**, 101–109.
Scangos, F. and Ruddle, F. H. (1981). *Gene* **14**, 1–4.
Schibler, U., Hagenbuchle, O., Wellauer, P. K. and Pittet, C. (1983). *Cell* **33**, 501–508.
Shimonkevitz, R., Luescher, B., Cerottini, J. C. and MacDonald, H. R. (1985). *J. Immunol.* **135**, 892–899.
Shinitzky, M. and Henkart, P. (1980). *Int. Rev. Cytol.* **60**, 121–147.
Sutherland, J., Mannoni, P., Rosa, F., Hatat, D., Turner, A. R. and Fellous, M. (1985). *Hum. Immunol.* **12**, 65–73.
Trinchieri, G. and Perussia, B. (1985). *Immunology Today* **6**, 131–134.

Virelizier, J. L., Perez, N., Arenzana-Seisdedos, F. and Devos, R. (1984). *Eur. J. Immunol.* **14**, 106, 108.
Walker, M. D., Edlund, T., Boulet, A. M. and Rutter, W. (1983). *Nature* (*London*) **306**, 557–559.
Wallach, D., Fellous, M. and Revel, M. (1982). *Nature* (*London*) **299**, 833–836.
Weber, J., Jelinck, W. and Darnell, J. E. Jr. (1977). *Cell* **10**, 611–617.
Wollman, E. E. and Kalil, J. (1983). *Tissue Antigens* **22**, 37–47.
Wong, G. H. W., Clark-Lewis, I., Mekimm-Bresckin, J. L. and Schrader, J. W. (1982). *Proc. Natl Acad. Sci. USA* **79**, 6989–6993.
Yoishie, O., Schmidt, H., Lengyel, P., Reddy, E. S. P., Morgan, W. R. and Weissman, S. M. (1984). *Proc. Natl Acad. Sci. USA* **81**, 649–653.

Cytotoxins (Tumour Necrosis Factor, Lymphotoxin and Others): Molecular and Functional Characteristics and Interactions with Interferons

DAVID WALLACH

Department of Virology, The Weizmann Institute of Science, Rehovot, Israel.

ABBREVIATIONS

The following abbreviations and synonyms will be used

ADCC = antibody-dependent cytotoxicity
CHI = cycloheximide
CTX = cytotoxins
DTH = delayed-type hypersensitivity
HA = haemagglutination units
IFN = interferon
IL-1 = interleukin 1
LPS = bacterial lypopolysaccharides
LT = lymphotoxin
mAb = monoclonal antibody
MHC = major histocompatibility complex
MP = mononuclear phagocytes

INTERFERON 7
ISBN 0 12 302256 8

NK = natural killer
NKCF = natural killer cytotoxic factor
PAGE = polyacrylamide gel electrophoresis
PBMC = peripheral-blood mononuclear leukocytes
PHA = phytohaemagglutinin
PMA = 4βphorbol-12-myristate-13-acetate
SDS = sodium dodecyl sulphate
TNF = tumour necrosis factor
VSV = vesicular stomatitis virus

I INTRODUCTION

Awareness of the anticellular activity of the interferons (IFNs), and of the existence of cytokines other than IFNs with anticellular activity, has developed in parallel. Initial studies on the anticellular effects of IFNs were with crude preparations (Pauker *et al.*, 1962). This raised doubts about whether IFN in these preparations did indeed mediate the observed effects, and not other, contaminating, cytokines. Conversely, the existence of cytokines, other than IFNs, with cytotoxic activity ('cytotoxins'—CTXs) has for quite a time been questioned in view of the fact that the crude preparations in which these mediators were detected. (Granger and Kolb, 1968; Ruddle and Waksman, 1968; Carswell *et al.*, 1975) did contain IFNs. With the purification of IFNs and, very recently, two CTXs—lymphotoxin and tumour necrosis factor (Aggarwal *et al.*, 1984, 1985; Haranaka *et al.*, 1985) it was confirmed that both the IFNs and the CTXs have their own anticellular activities. It was also observed that the two kinds of mediators may act in concert: their anticellular activities are synergistic; other effects of CTXs, besides their anticellular ones, are also potentiated by IFNs. Furthermore, IFNs promote the formation of CTXs, and CTXs can induce the formation of IFNs.

We are attempting now to throw light on the mechanisms which underlie these interrelationships of IFNs and CTXs and to understand their physiological significance. Our concepts on these subjects are still in a state of flux. In fact, even the terminology for the CTXs is still undefined and may have to remain so until we have a better idea of the extent of multiplicity and heterogeneity of the CTXs. In this review, I have tried to extract from the fragmentary information available as comprehensive an understanding as possible and to speculate on aspects in which there are still gaps in our knowledge. A suggestion made by Donald Metcalf (1975) may be appropriate to apply at this point: 'Remember that no matter how enthusiastic you may be about the significance of your observations, if your paper is re-read in 10 years' time, your original interpretation of the data will almost certainly be wrong, if not hilariously so.' It may take much less than 10 years in the field of CTX research.

This review focuses on those aspects of our knowledge of CTXs concerning the interrelationship between CTXs and IFNs. For a survey of other aspects of CTX research there are a number of useful reviews (Rosenau, 1980; Klostergaard *et al.*, 1981; Ruff and Gifford, 1981a; Ruddle *et al.*, 1983).

II THE CYTOTOXINS

A Terminology

There is at present some ambiguity in the terminology of the CTXs. Terms coined in the past for crude preparations of CTX have now been adopted for the purified proteins (Table I). Yet cytotoxic activities of the crude preparations cannot always be fully accounted for by those of the isolated proteins bearing the same name. Furthermore, we now know that there is a significant overlap in the kinds of CTXs present in crude preparations that were given differing names. To avoid misunderstanding, I have chosen to refer in this review to all crude preparations of the proteins by the general term cytotoxins, specifying when necessary the conditions of induction. (An exception is the term 'NKCF' which will be used here, as elsewhere, for describing the CTXs produced by NK cells in response to tumor cells.) The terms 'lymphotoxin' and 'TNF' will be applied solely in reference to the purified proteins.

Nevertheless, it may be useful to review briefly the various terms for the crude CTX preparations formerly in use, as a way of introducing some of the major milestones in CTX research. The term 'lymphotoxin' (LT) was coined for CTX preparations induced in lymphocyte cultures by mitogenic lectins and by antigens. These were first described by Granger and Kolb (1968) and by Ruddle and Waksman (1968). Later studies, primarily by G. Granger and his collaborators, demonstrated heterogeneity in physiochemical as well as in serological properties of PHA-induced CTXs. Differing fractions of such preparations, separated by gel filtration and by ion-exchange chromatography, have been termed 'LT-α, β and γ' for what appeared to be main size populations of the CTXs. LT-α1 denoted a subfraction of LT-α in DEAE-cellulose chromatography, and so on (*c.f.* Granger *et al.*, 1978).

Production of some cytotoxic factors also by cultured mononuclear phagocytes (MP) was noted quite some time ago (*cf.* Pincus, 1967). However, the first detection of that specific CTX we now call 'tumor necrosis factor' (TNF) can be traced to a study in 1975, describing induction of haemorrhagic necrosis in a transplantable methylcholanthrene-induced sarcoma by *in vivo* produced CTXs. These CTXs were induced by injecting mice with bacterial lipopolysaccharides (LPS) following priming with Bacillus-Calmette Guérin (Carswell *et al.*, 1975). Initially circumstantial evidence, and later serological

TABLE I Modes of Induction, Terms Used for Differing Preparations of CTXs and Identity of Concomitantly Formed IFNs

Producer cells	Inducing agents	Terms for crude preparations of induced CTXs	Terms for isolated CTXs	IFNs induced
T-cells (primarily Lyt-1^+)	T-cell mitogens (antigens; lectins; allogeneic cells; IL-2 . . .)	Lymphotoxins (LTs)	LT (or TNF-β) (and TNF-α?)	IFN-γ
Lymphoblastoid B cells	4β-phorbol-12-myristate-13-acetate (PMA)			
Mononuclear phagocytes	LPS; PMA; Sendai virus; Tumour cells.	Tumour necrosis factor (TNF)	TNF (or "Necrosin" or TNF-α or "cachectin")	IFN-α and β
NK cells	Tumour cells	Natural killer cytotoxic factor (NKCF)	(TNF ?)	IFN-α

examination (Männel *et al.*, 1980), affirmed the identity of these CTXs produced *in vivo* with those produced *in vitro* by cultured mononuclear phagocytes (MP).

More recent studies have demonstrated production of CTXs also by natural-killer (NK) cells, in response to certain tumour target cells; those CTX preparations were termed 'natural killer cytotoxic factors' (NKCF) (Wright and Bonavida, 1982).

B Characteristics of the Isolated CTXs.

Crude preparations of lymphotoxins, tumour necrosis factor and NKCF all contain IFNs. Since IFNs by themselves can exert cytostatic and cytotoxic activities, separating the two kinds of factors depends on first defining functional criteria whereby they differ from each other. The most evident difference between the two is that CTXs do not have the antiviral activity that characterizes the IFNs. In addition, clear differences can also be discerned in the way IFNs and CTXs exert their anticellular effects: killing of cells by IFNs, like all other effects of the IFNs, is dependent on synthesis of some proteins in the affected cell. On the other hand, cell killing by CTXs is found to be mediated independently of protein synthesis and, in fact, to be greatly potentiated by inhibitors of protein and of RNA synthesis. Furthermore, species-specificity to the extent observed in IFN function is not observed in the cytotoxic function of CTX preparations.

As shown in Fig. 1, which demonstrates separation of a CTX (TNF) from an IFN (IFN-γ) and separation of the mRNAs for the two proteins, these functional differences between CTXs and IFNs can allow specific detection of the one in the presence of the other. IFNs can be determined in the presence of CTXs by measuring the antiviral effect of the former, while CTXs can be specifically determined in the presence of IFN by measuring cytotoxic effects exerted in the presence of inhibitors of RNA or of protein synthesis. Alternatively, the cytotoxic activity of CTXs can be specifically determined in the presence of IFNs by using cells of a remote animal species which would not respond to the species-specific IFN effect (e.g. use of mouse L929 cells for detecting human TNF).

Two CTXs have recently been isolated—one, a glycoprotein with an M_r of about 25 Kd was isolated from preparations of CTXs produced by cells of a B-lymphoblastoid cell line (Aggarwal *et al.*, 1984) and the other, a non-glycosylated protein, with an M_r of about 17 Kd—from preparations of the CTXs induced in cells of a promyelocytic cell line (Aggarwal *et al.*, 1985a; Haranaka *et al.*, 1985). The two proteins turned out to be closely related in structure, so that while initially they were called lymphotoxin (LT) and tumour necrosis factor (TNF), it was suggested recently that they be named

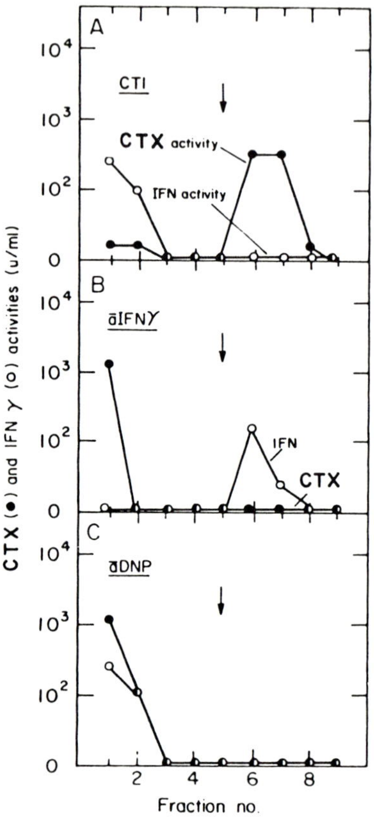
A
CTI
CTX activity
IFN activity
B
āIFNγ
IFN
CTX
C
āDNP
0
10²
10³
10⁴
2
4
6
8
Fraction no.
CTX (●) and IFN γ (○) activities (u/ml)

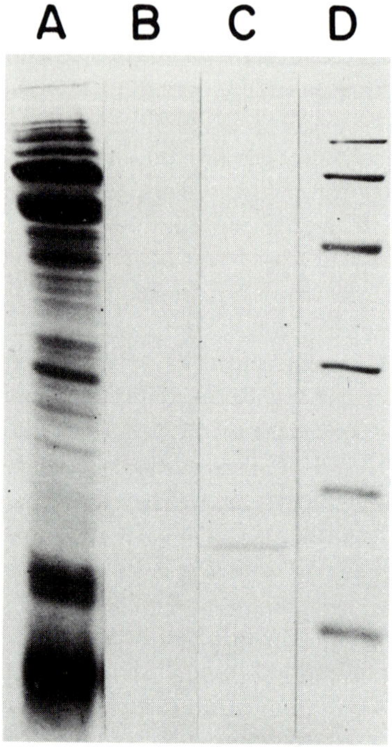
A
B
C
D

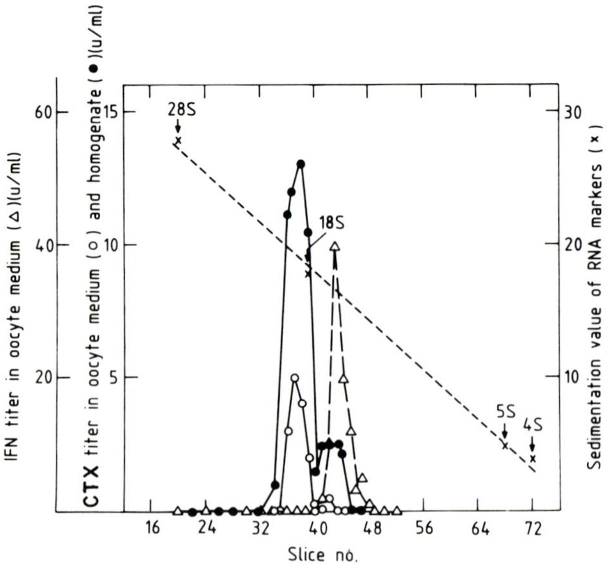
28S
18S
5S
4S
16
24
32
40
48
56
64
72
Slice no.
IFN titer in oocyte medium (Δ)(u/ml)
CTX titer in oocyte medium (○) and homogenate (●)(u/ml)
Sedimentation value of RNA markers (×)
20
40
60
5
10
15
30

TNF β and α respectively. The mouse homologue of TNF was initially called 'necrosin' (Kull and Cuatrecasas, 1984). This term was coined by Menkin (1943), for an *in vivo*, induced factor, recovered from pleural exudates of dogs injected with turpentine, that could induce cellular injury in animals resembling that observed in inflammation.

The amino acid sequence of LT and TNF, as established from analysis of the proteins themselves as well as from sequencing their complementary and genomic DNAs, were found to be remarkably homologous (Aggarwal *et al.*, 1984, 1985; Gray *et al.*, 1984; Pennica *et al.*, 1984; Shirai *et al.*, 1985; Wang *et al.*, 1985; Fransen *et al.*, 1985). By introducing gaps in the structure of LT, the two sequences can be aligned with an identity of 28% and with homology (including conservative changes) of 46% of their amino acids. Differences are largely confined to a single region in the molecules (residues 69–101 in TNF and 86–118 in LT). That 32-amino-acid region is, in TNF, confined by a disulfide bridge (between cysteins 69 and 101) which probably imposes on this sequence a loop structure separated from the rest of the molecule.

The similarity in structure between TNF and LT is reflected in their functions which, so far, appear to be indistinguishable. However, the differences in structure between the two proteins may yet be found to be functionally meaningful. The sequence homology between TNF and LT is significantly less than that between human and mouse TNF (Fransen *et al.*, 1985; Marmenout *et al.*, 1985; Pennica *et al.*, 1985). Almost complete homology (including conservative changes) in the amino acid sequences of TNF from the two sources is observed not only throughout the mature molecules but also in the structure of their leader portion, which in TNF is significantly longer (76 residues) than in LT (34 residues): it is encoded by exons distinct from those coding for most of the mature protein. The effective preservation,

---

Fig. 1. **(A)** and **(B)** Isolation of TNF by the use of a monoclonal antibody (mAb) to the protein (Hahn *et al.*, 1985). (C) Dissociation of the mRNAs for TNF and IFN-γ using the oocyte microinjection technique for determining translational activity of the two mRNAs (Wallach *et al.*, 1984).

(A) Fractionation of a cytokine preparation containing the two proteins using immunoadsorbents constructed with mAbs against TNF (A), IFN-γ (B) or dinitrophenyl (C). Bound proteins were eluted with 0.2 M NH_4OH (arrow).

(B) SDS/15%-PAGE of TNF purified by immunoadsorption. The crude preparation of the protein (A); NH_4OH-eluted fraction from the immunoadsorbent constructed with the anti-dinitrophenyl mAb (B); TNF purified on the mAb against this protein (C); molecular weight standards (94; 67; 43; 30; 20.1 and 14.4) (D).

(C) 1.2% agarose–methylmercuric hydroxide gel electrophoresis of poly$(A)^+$ RNA from stimulated human PBMC. RNA extracted from slices of the gel was microinjected into *Xenopus* oocytes and the level of cytotoxic activity in the oocyte homogenates (●) as well as the cytotoxic (○) and IFN activity (△) in the oocyte incubation media were determined 24 hours following microinjection.

TNF activity was determined by measuring cytotoxic effect on SV-80 cells in the presence of CHI and IFN-activity by determining reduction in the cytophatic effect of Vesicular stomatitis virus (VSV) on WISH cells.

through evolution, of parts of TNF differing from LT implies that these sequences are functionally important and that their alteration in the evolution of LT may be functionally meaningful.

At present it is not clear how many other CTXs there are besides TNF and LT. The recently described 'perphorins' are CTXs that appear to function quite differently from LT and TNF and are therefore likely to differ from these proteins in structure as well. The perphorins are components of cytoplasmic granules of cytotoxic T-lymphocytes and of NK cells. Upon interaction of the isolated granules or of the intact cytotoxic cells with membranes the proteins form, in a Ca^{2+}-dependent manner, tubular complexes that are inserted into the membranes and cause cytolysis (Podack (1985)). Purification of "perphorin" and initial characterization of its molecular properties have recently been reported (Young *et al.*, 1986).

There have been a few reports of purification of some other CTXs that apparently differ from TNF and LT (e.g. Ransom *et al.*, 1985; Rubin *et al.*, 1985). Moreover, some proteins of non leukocyte origin which exert cytostatic effects have also been isolated (e.g. cf. Roberts *et al.*, 1985). It is not yet known to what extent, if any, these proteins are structurally related to TNF and LT.

III CTX FORMATION AND ITS ENHANCEMENT BY IFN

A Production of CTXs and of IFN in Response to the Same Inducing Agents

A considerable number of agents were found to induce the production of CTXs. As demonstrated in Fig. 2, effective production of CTXs can be induced in human peripheral blood mononuclear cells (PBMC) by agents as different from each other as phytohaemagglutinin (PHA) and Sendai virus. These two agents induce the proteins by affecting different kinds of leukocytes. Sendai virus induces the production of CTXs in MP, while PHA induces CTXs by stimulating non-adherent mononuclear cells (apparently T-cells) (Table II). Other T cell mitogens—such as foreign antigens—also induce CTXs in T cells (Ruddle *et al.*, 1985). In addition, bacterial lipopolysaccharides induce CTXs in MP (Ruff and Glifford, 1981a); the diterpene tumour promotor 4-β-phorbol-12-myristate-13-acetate (PMA) induces CTXs in MP as well as in certain lymphoid B and T cell lines (Gifford *et al.*, 1984; Williamson *et al.*, 1983; Adolf, 1984) and tumour cells can induce CTXs both in MP and in NK cells (Männel, 1981; Wright and Bonavida, 1982). The main CTX found to be produced by MP is TNF, while lymphocytes were reported to produce primarily LT (Chroboczek-Kelker *et al.*, 1985).

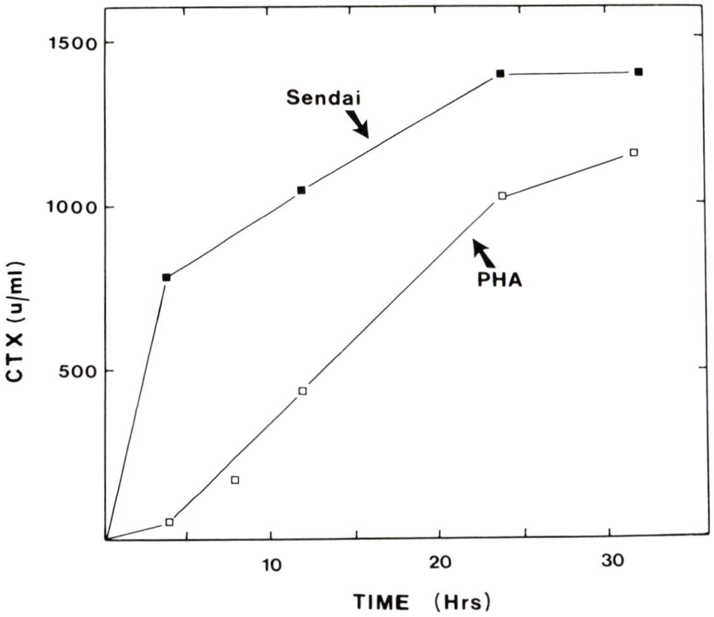

Fig. 2 Induction of CTXs in human PBMC (10^7 cells/ml) with Sendai virus (500 HA/ml) and with PHA (5 μg/ml) (Aderka *et al.*, 1986a).

TABLE II Differing Responsiveness of Mononuclear Phagocytes and of the Nonadherent Fraction of PBMC to Different Inducers of CTXs

Inducer	MP	Nonadherent PBMC (Primarily T-lymphocytes)
	CTX Yields (U/ml)	
None	10	< 5
PHA (5 μg/ml)	15	95
Con-A (20 μg/ml)	15	35
LPS (10 μg/ml)	30	< 5
PMA (5 ng/ml)	330	10
Sendai virus (500 HA/ml)	3000	15
LPS + PMA	2600	10

CTX induction (for 24 hours) by various agents, in fractionated human peripheral-blood mononuclear cells (PBMC) (Aderka *et al.*, 1986a).

Agents that stimulate T lymphocytes may, however, be found to induce significant production of TNF as well in cultures of PBMC, apparently through indirect stimulation of MP by the stimulated T cells (Aderka *et al.*, 1986a; Nedwin *et al.*, 1985). The identity of the CTXs comprising NKCF preparations is not yet clear. There have been preliminary reports suggesting that these preparations may contain TNF as well as CTXs that differ from TNF (Svedersky *et al.*, 1985a; Ortaldo *et al.*, 1985).

Those agents that induce production of CTXs in the various leukocytes also induce IFNs in the same cells (Table I): T cell mitogens induce in T cells the production of IFN-γ together with LT. Agents that stimulate MP to produce TNF also induce in these cells IFN-α and IFN-β, while in NK cells tumour cells induce the production of IFN-α as well as NKCF. Indeed, significant amounts of IFN would be detected in preparations of CTXs (see Matthews 1979; Ware and Granger, 1979).

B Enhancement of CTX Production by IFN

To find out if the IFNs produced with CTXs have a regulatory role in CTX induction, we have compared the efficiency of CTX production by PBMC pretreated with IFN-β to CTX production by untreated cells. No CTXs were induced as a result of treatment by IFN. However, when challenged by PHA, the IFN-treated cells produced CTXs at a significantly higher rate than untreated cells (Wallach and Hahn, 1983) (Fig. 4A). Furthermore, it could be shown, using antibodies to IFN, that production of CTXs by PHA-stimulated leukocytes that had not been pretreated by IFN was augmented, during prolonged incubation, by the IFN-γ produced *in situ* (Wallach *et al.*, 1983).

Enhancement of CTX production by IFN has turned out to be the rule for a variety of processes in which CTXs are formed, including the induction of CTXs in PBMC by antibody-coated cells IL-2, Concanavalin A (Con A), or staphylococcal enterotoxin A where, with the use of specific antibodies to TNF and LT it could be shown that production of both these CTXs were enhanced (Wallach *et al.*, 1983; Svedersky *et al.*, 1985b; Nedwin *et al.*, 1985). Production of TNF by mononuclear phagocytes in response to LPS and of NKCF by NK cells in response to tumour target cells was also found to be enhanced by IFN (Kildahl-Anderson *et al.*, 1985; Farram and Targan, 1983; Wright and Bonavida, 1983a; Steinhauer *et al.*, 1985). Furthermore, injection of IFN-γ into mice potentiated the production of TNF in subsequent injection of LPS (G. E. Gifford, and M. L. Lohmann-Matthes, personal communication). Augmentation *in vivo* of TNF production by IFN in man could be observed in patients with hairy-cell leukemia. The PBMC of these patients produce TNF poorly in response to stimulation *in vitro* by PHA, PMA or

Sendai virus. However, following a month of treatment by IFN-α, production of TNF in response to PHA increases, reaching close to normal values. This augmentation appears to reflect both increase in counts of MP and in responsiveness of the cells to induction of TNF (Aderka *et al.*, 1986b).

C Mechanisms Involved

There is inherent complexity in the processes of CTX induction and in their regulation. Within the CTX-producing cell, components and mechanisms at differing subcellular sites take part in the sequence of events that lead from the initial interaction of the cell with a CTX inducer to the eventual secretion of the CTXs. Furthermore, indirectly, mechanisms functioning outside the CTX-producing cell may also affect the formation of CTXs. Since CTX formation may be induced by cell-associated components (e.g. foreign antigens on the surface of cells), whose expression can be modulated, mechanisms functioning within such CTX-inducing cells may have a regulatory role in the production of CTXs. In addition, as discussed below, the production of CTXs may be affected by regulatory cytokines, whose own formation can be modulated by regulatory agents. There are thus multiple potential sites for regulation by IFN of the processes involved in CTX induction.

Direct information on mechanisms that participate in CTX production is scarce. However, based on indirect information I list below cellular activities and components likely to take part in the processes of CTX induction, in order to point out effects of IFN through which these processes can be modulated. These putative sites for regulation of CTX production by IFN, as well as the mode of regulation by IFN of CTX effects on cells, are depicted diagrammatically in Fig. 3.

1 Regulation of CTX formation at the level of CTX-producing cells

Since CTX-inducing agents are primarily extracellular, while the production of CTXs occurs within the cell, there are likely to be cell surface receptors or sensing mechanisms for these agents that initiate the production of CTXs. Such sensors are the T cell antigen receptors, which are probably involved in the induction of CTXs in T cells by antigens; the Fc receptor, which is likely to take part in induction of CTXs as part of antibody-dependent cytotoxicity (ADCC); membrane structures with which LPS interacts when inducing CTXs in MP; and others. We know very little about the nature of the intracellular mediating mechanisms that transduce the signal for CTX induction. Cyclic AMP, a mediator in many hormonal processes, is unlikely to be involved, at least not as a positive signal, since agents that increase cyclic

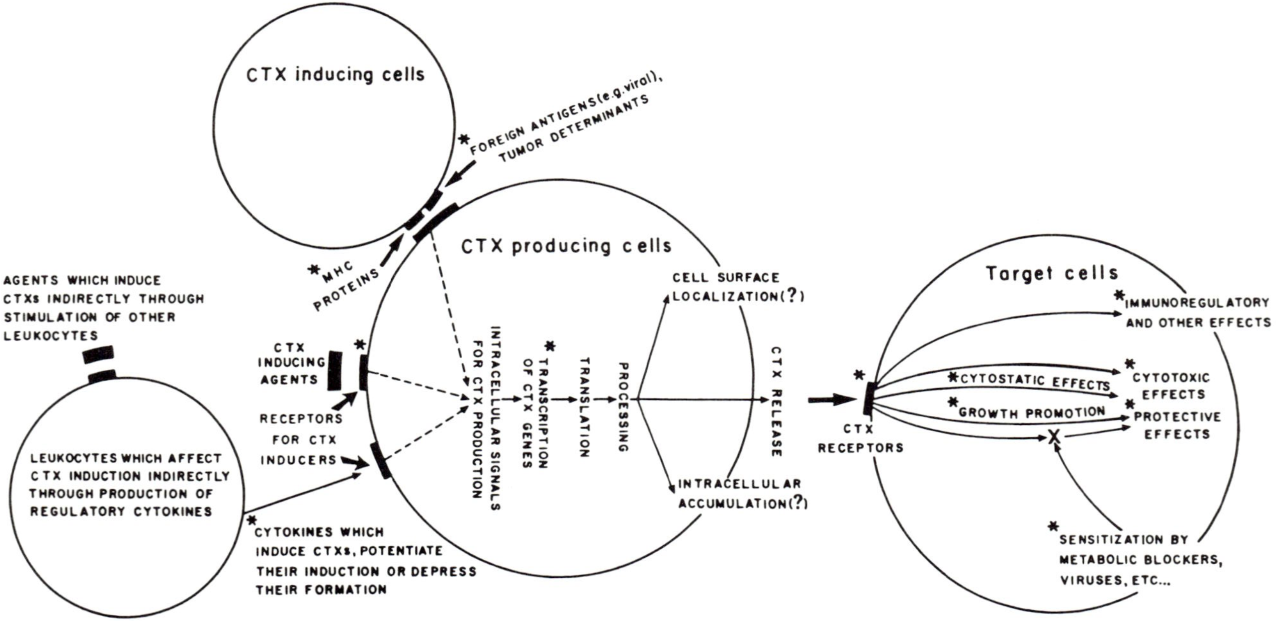

Fig. 3 Putative points of regulation by IFN (denoted by asterisks) in processes of CTX formation and in the response of target cells to the effect of CTXs.

AMP level in leukocytes have been found to suppress the formation of CTXs (Wallach *et al.*, 1983).

One may speculate, on the basis of effects of calcium modulating agents on the production of CTXs by lymphocytes, and on the basis of the ability of the diterpene ester PMA to induce CTXs in MP and in lymphocytes (Wallach *et al.*, 1983; Williamson *et al.*, 1983; Gifford *et al.*, 1984 and Adolf, 1984), that calcium fluxes or protein phosphorylation initiated by protein kinase C (known to be activated by PMA) play a role as mediating signals in the production of CTXs by these cells.

So far, the only intracellular event in CTX formation monitored with the use of a molecular probe is the transcription of CTX genes. mRNAs for TNF and LT could be detected in CTX-producing cells by hybridization to a cDNA probe (Gray *et al.*, 1984 and Svederksy *et al.*, 1985b) as well as by injection of the RNA into *Xenopus* oocytes, where it could be translated to biologically active TNF molecules (Wallach *et al.*, 1984, and Fig. 1C). With either of these techniques, significant increases in CTX mRNA upon CTX induction could be detected, indicating regulation of CTX formation on the level of synthesis, processing or degradation of mRNA (Wallach *et al.*, 1984 and Svedersky *et al.*, 1985b).

Little information is available as to the nature of post-translational events in CTX induction. In the formation of TNF, post-translational processing, involving the removal of a long signal peptide, has to occur prior to release of these molecules from the cell. The site and mechanism of this processing have not been identified as yet. Indirect evidence based on the effects of protein synthesis and cytoskeletal inhibitors on the release of CTXs by lectin-stimulated lymphocytes, and localization studies using antibodies raised against partially purified preparations of these CTXs, were interpreted as suggesting that CTXs can accumulate in lymphocytes both intracellularly and on the cell surface (see Hiserodt *et al.*, 1977, 1979).

Evidence for intracellular accumulation of NKCF in NK cells has also been presented based on detection of NKCF-like activity in homogenates of these cells (Wright and Bonavida, 1983a). The presence of NKCF in intracellular stores is also indicated by the ability of antibodies to preparations of the large granules of NK cells to block the cytotoxic activity of NKCF (Ortaldo *et al.*, 1985). Furthermore, antibodies raised against partially purified MP-produced CTXs were shown to interact with intracellular proteins in mononuclear phagocytes (Kildahl-Andersen *et al.*, 1985). The use of monospecific antibodies to CTXs should now generate more reliable and detailed information on the subcellular localization of CTXs within CTX-producing cells and on the mechanisms of their release.

In an attempt to clarify the IFN-regulated mechanisms that take part in the enhancement of CTX formation by lectin-stimulated PBMC pretreated with IFN, we first questioned whether the IFN-induced changes in this case occur in the CTX-producing cells themselves or are the result of a secondary effect, due to altered production of regulatory cytokines secreted by some leukocytes within the heterogeneous population of the PBMC. Preliminary data (Fig. 4) suggest that lectin-stimulated PBMC secrete cytokines, distinct from IFN (or CTXs), that enhance CTX formation as effectively as IFN. When applied on PBMC, IFN-free preparations of these cytokines did not induce production of CTXs (except at significantly higher concentrations than used in our experiments). However, on subsequent stimulation by PHA, PBMC treated at the lower concentrations of cytokines responded much more rapidly than non-treated cells in release of CTXs. In fact, this occurred just as rapidly as CTX release from IFN-pretreated cells (Fig. 4A).

The amounts of cytokines responsible for this effect could be estimated indirectly by determining how effectively the cytokine preparations enhanced CTX formation (Fig. 4B). Thus, it was shown that IFN-pretreated leukocytes produce more of these cytokines than cells that were not treated by IFN (Fig. 4C). Although the cytokines responsible for this effect have not yet been identified, the findings in this experimental system indicate that IFN-induced enhancement of CTX formation, at least in part, indirectly reflects enhanced formation of cytokines which themselves have a stimulatory effect on CTX formation. This complex mode of regulation by IFN may result in enhanced, cascade-like, stimulatory effect.

CTX formation and function may also be modulated by suppressive factors. The delayed type hypersensitivity (DTH) response, which probably involves CTX formation (see below), can be effectively blocked by suppressor cells. The decreased activity of suppressor cells, observed following treatment by IFN (Knop *et al.*, 1982) may further contribute to an increase in formation of CTXs.

Regulatory cytokines may function also as direct inducers of CTXs. Interleukin-2 was reported to induce effective production of both TNF and LT in cultures of PBMC (Svedersky *et al.*, 1985b; Nedwin *et al.*, 1985). IFN may increase the formation of interleukin-2 by enhancing the production of interleukin-1 and thus indirectly potentiate CTX production.

Modulation of production of regulatory cytokines is likely to contribute to a significant extent to the effect of IFN on formation of CTXs in cultures of mixed populations of leukocytes, where the differing kinds of mononuclear leukocytes indeed have marked regulatory effects on each other through the action of cytokines they secrete. To find out whether direct effects of IFN on CTX-producing cells may also contribute to the enhancement of CTX formation, we have sought to examine this regulation in a simpler experimental system—a homogeneous population of CTX-producing cells of cultured lines. Preliminary results from a study on the effect of IFN on the production

TABLE III Increase in Production of CTXs by U937 Cells Following Treatment by IFN, TNF or a Crude Leukocyte-produced Cytokine Preparation.

Preincubation	CTX yield (U/ml)		
	no inducing agents	LPS	Sendai virus
–	< 5	< 5	< 5
PMA	10	180	125
rIFN-γ	< 5	< 5	< 5
PMA + IFN-γ	35	500	625
PMA + TNF	10	440	N.T.*
PMA + TNF + IFN-γ	40	1030	N.T.
PMA + crude leukocyte cytokines	N.T.	3130	N.T.

U937 cells (10^6 cells/ml) in samples of 2 ml were incubated in 18 mm tissue culture wells for 24 hours with the agents indicated in the first column, then rinsed, brought to 1 ml and incubated further for 24 hours either alone or with LPS or with Sendai virus. Yields of CTXs in the cultures were then determined by measuring cytotoxic effect on CHI sensitized L132 cells. PMA was applied at 5 ng/ml, rIFN-γ at 1000 U/ml, TNF (native; homogeneously purified on the CT-1 mAb) at 100 U/ml, crude leukocyte cytokines (see below) at 0.2 μg/ml, LPS at 10 μg/ml and Sendai virus at 500 HA/ml. Leukocyte cytokines were induced in PBMC by 36 hours' stimulation with PMA (5 ng/ml) and Con-A (20 μg/ml), then concentrated by adsorption to controlled- pore glass and treated at pH 2.0 as described in the legend to Fig. 4. No IFN or CTX activity could be detected in this kind of preparation (unpublished observations).
*N.T.—not tested.

of CTXs by the human histiocytic lymphoma U937 cells are presented in Table III. Although unable to produce CTXs under normal growth conditions, the U937 cells do produce CTXs (primarily TNF) when induced to differentiate with PMA, and produce CTXs to an even greater extent when further treated either with LPS or with Sendai virus. As shown in Table III, IFN-γ enhances formation of the CTXs by the U937 cells. Although even in this case an indirect effect of IFN through induction of "autokines", which the U937 cells both produce and respond to, cannot be ruled out, it seems more likely that IFN enhances the production of CTXs in the U937 cells by inducing changes in cellular mechanisms directly involved in the process of CTX formation. Effects of regulatory cytokines other than IFN on CTX production may also be studied in the U937 cells. TNF itself potentiates the production of CTXs (actually its own production) in these cells, and that potentiation effect is additive to the effect of IFN-γ. Crude preparations of leukocyte-produced cytokines, free of both IFN and TNF, also have very strong potentiation effects on the production of CTXs by those cells (Table III).

Among the various components and mechanisms within the CTX-producing cell whose alteration by IFN may result in augmented production of the CTXs, one may first point out two specific receptors involved in these

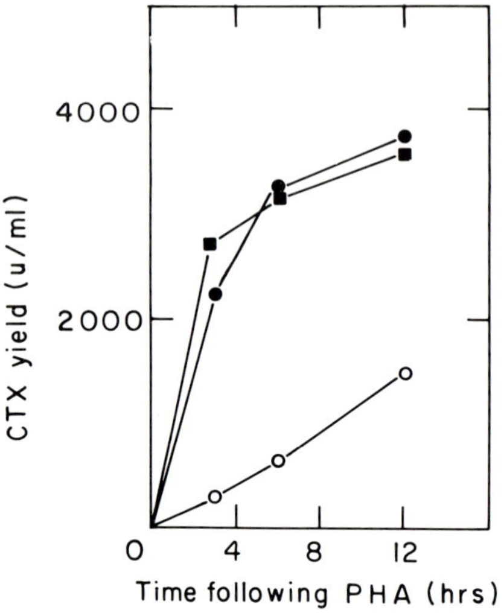

4000
2000
CTX yield (u/ml)
0
4
8
12
Time following PHA (hrs)

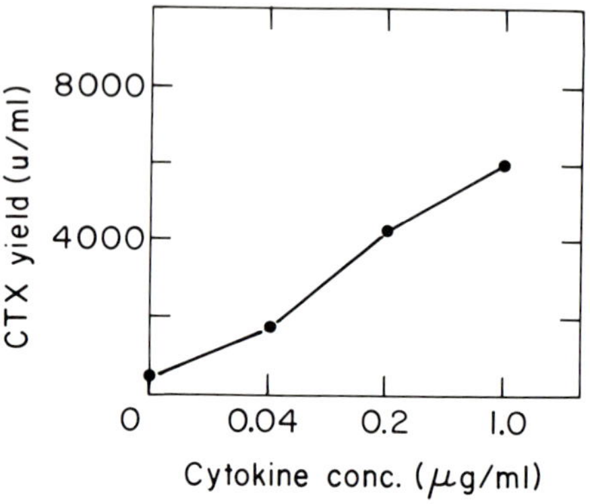

8000
4000
CTX yield (u/ml)
0
0.04
0.2
1.0
Cytokine conc. (μg/ml)

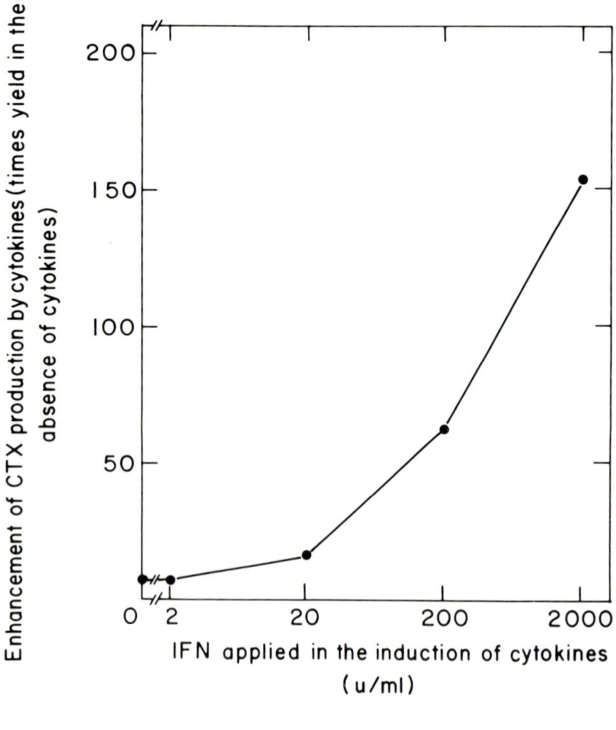

200
150
100
50
Enhancement of CTX production by cytokines (times yield in the absence of cytokines)
0
2
20
200
2000
IFN applied in the induction of cytokines (u/ml)

processes: the Fc receptor, whose increase by IFN may contribute to the augmented production of CTXs in antibody-dependent cytotoxic reactions, and the IL-2 receptor, which is also increased by IFN and which is likely to be involved in the induction of CTXs by T cell mitogens as well as by IL-2 itself. Recent findings by Sverdersky *et al.* (1985b) are consistent with the idea that transcription of mRNAs for CTXs is also enhanced by IFN. The level of mRNA for this CTX, in PBMC stimulated by IL-2 to produce CTXs, was estimated with the use of a cDNA probe for LT. In non-stimulated PBMC the concentration of mRNA for LT was below the level of detection; however, following treatment by IL-2, significant accumulation of the mRNA could be observed. In correlation with the effect of IFN on the production of LT itself, the mRNA for this protein did not increase on treatment by IFN-γ alone; but IFN treatment did enhance significantly the increase in mRNA observed on subsequent treatment with IL-2.

Fig. 4 IFN-induced increases in the production of CTXs and of cytokines which enhance CTX formation. (**A**) Kinetics of CTX production by PBMC in response to stimulation by PHA following pretreatment by IFN-α (1000 U/ml) (●) or by IFN-free leukocyte-produced crude cytokine preparation (0.2 μg/ml) (■), compared to CTX production in PBMC not pretreated by IFN nor by cytokines (○). (**B**) Titration of the stimulatory effect of the cytokine preparation on production of CTXs by PBMC in response to 6 hours' stimulation with PHA. (**C**) IFN-induced increase in production of the cytokines which enhance CTX formation.

PBMC isolated from freshly donated blood on a Ficoll-Hypaque cushion, were suspended in MEM-alpha medium at a concentration of 10^7 cells/ml, incubated for 12 hours with IFN or with the cytokines and then rinsed and treated with PHA-P (5 μg/ml). Cytotoxic activity in the culture medium was determined with the use of CHI-sensitized SV80 cells. The cytokine preparations were produced by treating PBMC for 12 hours with IFN-α (2000 U/ml in A, B and at varying concentrations in C) then rinsing the cells 3 times and applying Concanavalin A (Con-A 20 μg/ml) for 24 hours (6 hours in C). In A and B these cytokine preparations were concentrated by adsorption to controlled pore glass, eluted with 0.5 M tetramethylammonium chloride, further concentrated by ultrafiltration and incubated for 12 hours at pH 2.0. The ConA was eliminated in the adsorption to controlled pore glass. Acidification resulted in complete loss of IFN and of CTX activity of the cytokine preparation with no decrease in the effectiveness by which the cytokines enhanced CTX formation. Depletion of IFN-γ by applying these cytokine preparations on an immunoadsorbent constructed from a monoclonal antibody against that IFN did not decrease the effectiveness by which those cytokines augmented production of CTXs either. Inclusion of 50 mM α-methyl-D-mannopyranoside during CTX induction, to interfere with the function of any residual Con A, did not decrease the enhancement of CTX formation. Protein concentration in the crude cytokine preparation was about 1 μg/ml of leukocyte culture. In C, the preparations of cytokines (produced by cells pretreated with various concentrations of IFN-α and then stimulated for 6 hours with Con A) were not concentrated on controlled pore glass but just brought to pH 2.0 and 12 hours later returned to pH 7.0. The preparations were then applied at a dilution of 1 : 5 on PBMC in the presence of α-methyl-D-mannopyranoside (50 mM). The cells were incubated with the lymphokines for 12 hours and, after rinsing, for 6 further hours with PHA-P (5 μg/ml), yields of CTXs were determined. Yields of CTXs in the absence of pretreatment by cytokines were 68 U/ml in B and 11 U/ml in C. Electrophoretically pure native IFN-α was used in all experiments (unpublished observations).

2 Regulation at the level of CTX inducing cells

Additional potential sites for regulation by IFN can be discerned in those processes for CTX production in which the inducing agents are cells—cells which present foreign antigens on their surface and which induce CTXs in T lymphocytes, and tumour cells that induce CTXs in NK cells and in mononuclear phagocytes. The role of IFN in the production of CTXs by antigen-stimulated T cells has not, to my knowledge, yet been examined. In theory though, we may expect, that IFN will effectively modulate these processes of CTX production by inducing two kinds of changes: increase in major hystocompatibility (MHC) proteins, and the antiviral effect, neither when induced in the CTX-producing T cells but in the cells that present the stimulating antigens to the T-cells.

As in other processes of antigen-induced T cell activation, in the induction of CTXs in T cells, antigens have to be presented in association with the MHC proteins. This refers not only to cell-associated foreign antigens, but also to soluble antigens, since these are recognized by T cells only after being processed (primarily by MP) and exposed on the surface of the processing cell in association with MHC proteins.

Of the two major classes of the MHC proteins (Class I proteins HLA-A, -B, -C in man and H2-K and -D in mouse, and Class II proteins including HLA-DR in man and Ia in mouse), it seems that the class II proteins primarily take part in CTX induction. After fractionation of T cells, most cells capable of producing CTXs in response to antigens were Lyt-1^+ cells, known to recognize antigens in the context of the class II MHC proteins. Little CTX induction could be detected in the Lyt-2^+ cells, which recognize antigens associated with the class I MHC proteins (Eardley *et al.*, 1980; Tite *et al.*, 1985). IFNs, most notably, IFN-γ, enhance synthesis of the MHC proteins, particularly the class II MHC proteins (Lindahl *et al.*, 1974; Wallach, *et al.*, 1982; Basham and Merigan, 1983).

In a variety of cells, synthesis of the class II MHC proteins may, in fact, be observed only upon treatment by IFN-γ. IFN may in this way greatly promote antigen-induced CTX production. However, IFN may suppress induction of CTXs by antigens when these are virus-derived. This may not be an exceptional situation, since infecting viruses are probably the most common physiological source of cell-associated foreign antigens. Many viruses, however, do not respond to the antiviral effect; cell surface expression of viral antigen may even be found to be increased by IFN (Chang *et al.*, 1977).

On the whole, the combined effects of IFN on the MHC antigens and on the expression of viral antigens on the cell surface may be expected to result in decreased CTX induction by virus-infected cells whenever IFN suppresses replication of the virus, and in enhanced induction of CTXs by infected cells that fail to respond to the antiviral effect of IFN.

There is evidence that in the induction of CTXs in NK cells, too, IFN has a regulatory role at the level of the CTX-inducing cells. Mouse Yac cells, which can induce the production of NKCF, become less effective inducers when treated by IFN (Wright and Bonavida, 1983b). That observation is consistent with prior studies showing that IFNs, most notably IFN-γ, can suppress NK cytotoxicity by inducing resistance to killing in the target cells (Trinchieri and Santoli, 1978; Wallach, 1983). There is as yet no information on the molecular nature of these IFN-induced changes in NK-target cells or on the nature of the target structures for NK-cells in general.

IV CTX EFFECTS AND THEIR POTENTIATION BY IFN

A CTX Effects

1 Cytotoxic and cytostatic effects

In most studies on the cytotoxic effect of CTXs, the target cells have been L929 cells, which are particularly sensitive. From the limited characterization of the effect of CTXs on other cells, it appears that there is a wide spectrum of cells that are potentially sensitive to CTXs. However, in most of these cells the cytotoxic effect is rather slow, occurring in incubation for several days. A rapid cytotoxic effect, occurring within a few hours of CTX application, would not be observed unless the cells had been sensitized in some way. Such sensitization can be achieved by treating cells with metabolic blockers such as actinomycin D, cycloheximide (CHI), mitomycin-c, O-dinitrophenyl or sodium azide (Williams and Granger, 1973; Rosenau *et al.*, 1973; Ruff and Gifford, 1981b; Wallach, 1984, unpublished observations). It can also be induced by x-irradiation or by infection of the CTX-treated cells with certain viruses (Eifel *et al.*, 1979; Aderka *et al.*, 1985; and Figs 5 and 6).

Cells of several lines, including some that are quite resistant to the cytotoxicity of CTXs, can be found to respond to CTXs by arrest of cell growth. The relation of this cytostatic effect of CTXs to the cytotoxic activity is not clear. Possibly growth arrest by these proteins is, in many cases, an early reflection of cellular changes that eventually result in cell death. However, at least in some cells, growth arrest by CTXs may reflect specific inhibition of growth-related functions, as indicated by the fact that it results in accumulation of cells in specific stages of the cell cycle. Thus L929 cells were reported to respond to TNF in an arrest at G_2 (Darzynkiewicz *et al.*, 1984), and B16

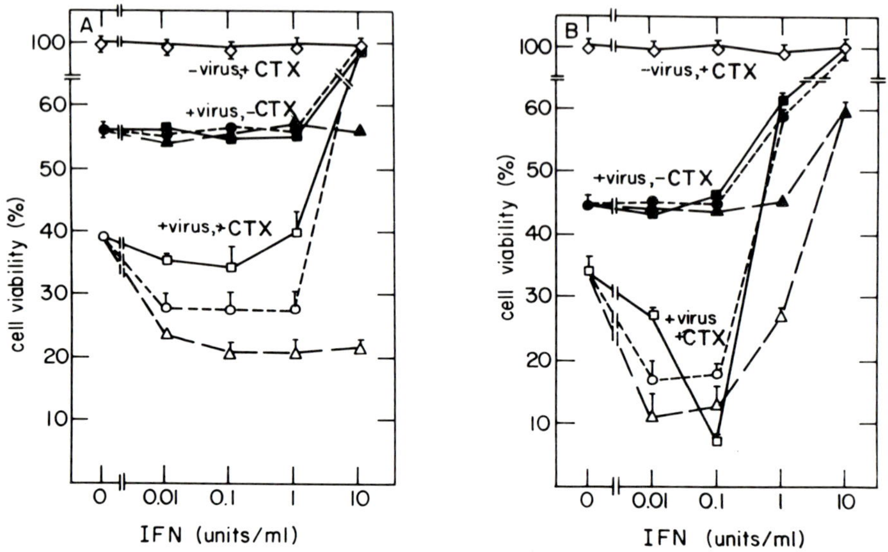

Fig. 5 IFN effects on the cytotoxicity of CTXs in SV80 cells (**A**) and in HeLa cells (**B**), IFN-α (○, ●), IFN-β (□, ■), and IFN-γ (△, ▲) were applied at the indicated concentrations prior to infection by VSV (solid symbols) or infection by VSV followed by application of CTX (6 U/ml, open symbols) or application of CTXs alone (6 U/ml, for the three types of IFN, ◇) (see note in Fig. 6 on the way the CTXs were induced). Note the enhancement of cell-killing at low concentrations of IFN as opposed to the protective effect of IFN at higher concentrations (Aderka *et al.*, 1985).

melanoma cells responded to purified LT, and more effectively to LT plus IFN-γ, in an arrest at the G_0/G_1 phase (Lee *et al.*, 1984). Indeed, there is preliminary evidence that transcription of the c-*myc* oncogene is in certain tumour cells, effectively turned off by TNF (Yarden, A., Wallach, D. and Kimchi, A. submitted).

2 *Protective and cell growth promoting effects*

Some of the molecular changes observed in cells treated by CTX are inconsistent with the cytotoxic and cytostatic functions of these proteins. Rather than interfering with viable functions of the cells, CTXs have been found to induce an increase in RNA, protein and lipid synthesis (Rosenau, 1980; Ostrove and Gifford, 1979). Furthermore, in cells resistant to the cytotoxic effect of CTXs, these proteins could even be found to stimulate cell multiplication (Sugarman, *et al.*, 1985; Fiers *et al.*, 1986; Vilček *et al.*, 1986). As discussed below, it appears that these "constructive" effects of CTXs in part reflect repair mechanisms that counteract the cytotoxic activity of these proteins, thus preventing non-selective cell destruction. It also seems possible

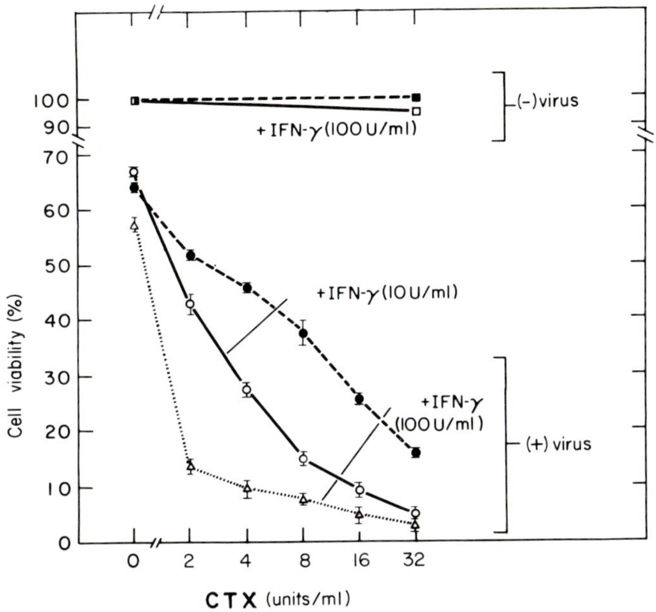

Fig. 6 Enhancement by IFN-γ of CTX cytotoxicity in VSV-infected SV80 cells. The cytotoxic effect of CTXs at various concentrations in VSV-infected cells (●) and its further enhancement by treating these cells with IFN-γ (10 U/ml) (○) or 100 U/ml (△)) 16 hours prior to infection is shown in comparison to the resistance to the CTXs observed in uninfected cells (■) even when treated with IFN-γ (□). The CTXs used in the experiments described in Figs 5 and 6 were crude preparations of CTXs induced by PHA in PBMC, partially purified by adsorption to controlled pore glass and fully depleted of IFN-γ by the use of a monoclonal antibody (Aderka *et al.*, 1985). Selective cytotoxicity against VSV infected cells and its augmentation by IFN could similarly be observed with use of pure TNF.

that these CTX effects contribute to repair on the multicellular level, namely to the increased cell growth necessary for healing the damage in necrotic areas, where at an earlier stage CTX effects have led to the death of cells.

3 *CTXs as pleiotropic mediators*

Apart from effects on cell growth and viability, TNF and LT have recently been found to exert a variety of other effects on cell function. Some of these are immunoregulatory effects; primarily effects on functions related to immune cytolysis. LT was reported to induce in granulocytes enhanced ADCC and phagocytic activities (Shalaby, *et al.*, 1985a) and TNF to increase ADCC activity in the U937 hystiocytic lymphoma cells (Shalaby, *et al.*, 1985b); it also enhances the production of CTXs by those cells (Table III). There is some evidence that TNF can promote the differentiation of cytotoxic T lymphocytes (cf. Fiers, *et al.*, 1986). Furthermore, it may enhance cell-killing by cytotoxic T lymphocytes through effects on the target cells: TNF increases the synthesis and cell surface expression of Class I MHC antigens (Collins, *et al.*, 1986) and, according to a preliminary report, also of Class II antigens (Chang and Lee, 1985). Cells that have been exposed to TNF may, therefore, be more effectively recognized by the MHC-restricted cytotoxic T lymphocytes.

Quite a different role for TNF was revealed in the recent identification of TNF with the "cachectin"—a cytokine which suppresses in adipocytes the activity of lipoprotein lipase and also induces in these cells a decrease of mRNAs for some other proteins involved in the differentiated function of the adipocyte (Beutler, *et al.*, 1985a; Torti, *et al.*, 1985). Apparently that effect of TNF contributes to the defence against disease by assuring the availability of lipids for rapid use. However, when induced for prolonged duration the "cachectin" effect of TNF may result in an excessive and dangerous weight loss (cachexia).

That TNF can mediate some deleterious effects in diseases is also indicated by a recent study showing that injected antibodies to TNF reduce in mice the lethal effect of bacterial endotoxins. This indicates that TNF has a causative role in bacterially-induced septic shock (Beutler *et al.*, 1985b).

Since this review was submitted for publication (15 November) until to date (June 1986) many additional effects of TNF on cell functions have been revealed. Quite an unexpected finding, derived both from the studies on TNF and from studies on interleukin-1 (IL-1), is that these two cytokines, which bare no similarity of structure and apparently function through binding to distinct receptors, affect cell function in quite a similar manner. IL-1 can actually be regarded as a cytotoxin-certain tumour cells are killed by IL-1 as effectively as by LT (Onozaki, *et al.*, 1985), IL-1 also shares the ability of TNF to stimulate growth of fibroblasts (Schmidt, *et al.*, 1982). Some other examples of the similarity in function of TNF and IL-1 are: (1) Induction, by both, of the synthesis of collagenase and of prostaglandin E_2, in fibroblasts (Dayer, *et al.*, 1984, 1985); (2) The "cachectin"-lime activity (suppression of lipoprotein lipase in adipocytes) found to be mediated, not only by TNF but also by IL-1 (Beutler and Cerami, 1985); (3) Activation of osteoclasts by the two (Dewhirst, *et al.*, 1985; Bertolini, *et al.*, 1986), and (4) Induction in endothelial cells of increased adhesivity to granulocytes and of synthesis of a cell surface protein which probably is involved in that adherence (Gamble, *et al.*, 1985; Schleimer and Rutledge, 1986; Pober, *et al.*, 1986). Particularly interesting from the point of view of IFN research is the finding that both IL-1 and TNF induce in fibroblasts the synthesis of a specific IFN (IFN-β_2) (Content, *et al.*, 1985; Kohase, *et al.*, 1986). According to preliminary reports, TNF induces synthesis of an IFN also in PBMC (Wong and Goeddel, 1985).

B IFN-induced Enhancement of CTX Function

The cytotoxic and cytostatic effects of CTXs and those of IFNs are exerted synergistically. An IFN-induced increase in anticellular activities of CTXs could be observed with crude CTX preparations and with purified TNF and LT (Williams and Bellanti, 1983; Williamson *et al.*, 1983; Wallach *et al.*, 1983; Stone-Wolff *et al.*, 1984; Lee *et al.*, 1984) as well as with preparations of NKCF (Wright and Bonavida, 1983b; Steinhauer *et al.*, 1985). Furthermore, immunoregulatory effects of TNF and LT were also reported to be potentiated by IFN (Shalaby *et al.*, 1985a, b).

Yet, even though IFN appears generally to potentiate the function of CTXs, it has so far not been found to interfere with selectivity in this function by inducing responsiveness to CTXs in cells that in the absence of IFN are completely unresponsive to these proteins. An example of a situation in which IFN potentiates CTX activity without decreasing its selectivity is presented in Figs 5 and 6 in which the cytotoxic effect of IFN-free CTX preparations in SV-80 and HeLa cells is quantitatively analysed, comparing cells that were infected by VSV to uninfected cells. Under normal growth conditions the cells are quite resistant to killing by CTXs but they do respond to the cytotoxic effect following infection by the virus (cf. Fig. 6, curves ■ and ●). IFN is found to potentiate killing of the infected cells but not to impose vulnerability to this cytotoxic effect on the uninfected cells (cf. Fig. 6, curves □ and △). Since, at antiviral concentrations, IFN suppressed replication of the virus, an IFN-induced increase in killing of the infected cells could only be observed at sub-antiviral concentrations. At higher IFN concentrations, suppression of virus replication by IFN resulted in resurgence of the resistance to the effect of the CTXs (compare, in Fig. 5B, the enhancement of killing of HeLa cells by IFN-γ at 0.01 U/ml to the protection from killing when the IFN concentration was 10 U/ml).

C Mechanisms Involved

Radioactively tagged TNF and LT bind to high-affinity sites on the surface of cells; the number of binding sites range from undetectable levels to as much as 18,000 per cell, depending on the cell line (Hass *et al.*, 1985; Kull *et al.*, 1985; Tsujimoto *et al.*, 1985, 1986; Israel *et al.*, 1986). Using bifunctional cross-linking agents, specific cell surface proteins could be observed to which TNF bind, forming conjugates with M_r of about 75 and 92 Kd (Fig. 7 and Kull *et al.*, 1985).

These findings provide direct evidence for the long-suspected existence of cell surface receptors for CTXs. A clear distinction can now be made between those CTXs that function through binding to specific receptors and other

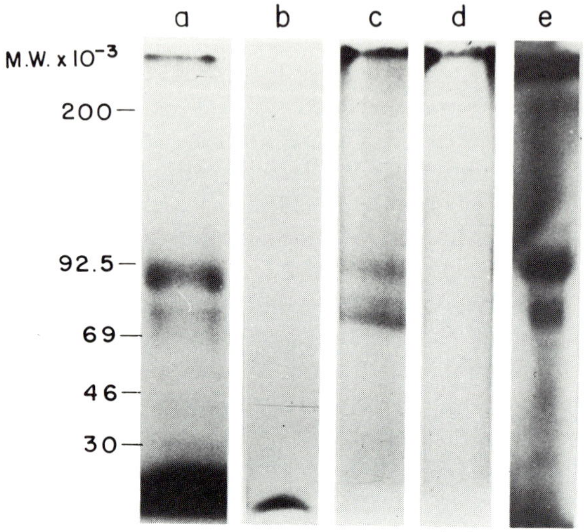

Fig. 7 Characterization of the receptors to human TNF on human U937 (a, b) and KG-1 (c–e) cells by their cross-linking to ^{125}I-TNF. **a**, **b**, **e**: cross-linking with disuccinimidyl suberate (in b-excess nonlabelled TNF was included during incubation with the labelled protein). **c**, **d**: cross-linking with the bifunctional agent dithiobis succinimidyl propionate which is cleavable with β-mercaptoethanol; analysis in the absence (c) and presence (d) of β-mercaptoethanol. Cells were incubated for 2 hours with ^{125}I-TNF (100 U/ml), which was radio-iodinated by the chloramine-T method. They were then washed, treated with the cross-linking agents and extracted with a buffer containing 2% Triton X-100. The extracts were analysed by SDS/7.5%-PAGE followed by autoradiography. The heavy radioactive band at the bottom of lane a is free TNF (Israel *et al.*, 1986).

cytotoxic proteins, also present in crude CTX preparations, that kill cells via enzymic activity (e.g. arginase or protease (Currie, 1978; Adams, 1980)). A third mode of cell-killing by leukocyte-produced proteins is exemplified in the function of the 'perphorins' (see Section II (B)) which, like the C_9 component of the complement, are believed to kill cells by forming channel-like structures in cell membranes, apparently with no prior interaction with any receptor protein.

The nature of the mechanisms activated by occupation of the TNF receptor, and which eventually lead to the functional changes induced by the CTXs, remains obscure. Similarly to cell surface receptors for many other agonists, the receptors for TNF are taken up into the cell after becoming occupied and the CTXs bound to these receptors are then degraded, apparently in lysosomes (Tsujimoto *et al.*, 1985). Clearly this uptake process has no role in the cytotoxic effect, as cytotoxicity can be effectively induced in the presence of sodium azide, which fully blocks the uptake (unpublished results). Neither does it appear that the cytotoxic effect is dependent on synthesis of any protein or RNA in the target cell, since it occurs in the presence of azide, CHI or actinomycin D; these agents actually potentiate the cytotoxic effect of CTXs. The fact that the cytotoxic effect of CTXs is exerted in the presence of inhibitors of RNA, protein and ATP synthesis, also implies that the CTXs themselves do not possess such a general inhibitory capacity and that their cytotoxic function reflects another mode of action. Specific RNA and protein species do decrease in response to TNF, apparently owing to suppressed synthesis of these molecules (Torti *et al.*, 1985), but TNF and LT have also been found to induce an increase in the synthesis of cellular RNA, proteins and lipids (Rosenau 1980; Ostrove and Gifford 1979).

Thus, as in the function of various other regulatory cytokines, we are faced in the function of CTXs with transduction of information from the receptors for these proteins to the interior of the cell, in a so far unknown fashion, resulting in altered synthesis of specific species of RNA and protein molecules and yet those effects are apparently distinct from those participating in the cytotoxic effect of the CTXs. Actually, as mentioned above, it has been suggested that the enhancement of synthesis of RNA, protein and lipid by CTXs has a role in counteracting the cytotoxic effects which the CTXs themselves induce (Rosenau, 1980). The fact that metabolic inhibitors such as CHI and actinomycin D, which are likely to interfere with CTX-induced increases in anabolic activities, sensitize cells to the cytotoxic effect, is consistent with a protective role for these CTX-induced changes. In further support for the idea that CTXs activate mechanisms in cells that counteract their cytotoxicity, we have found that, within a short time after application of CTXs, cells become less responsive to sensitization by CHI (Fig. 8).

Such induction of resistance to CTX by the CTX itself could be observed with purified TNF (Hahn *et al.*, 1985) as well as with partially purified preparations of LT, free of TNF, the two kinds of preparations inducing mutual resistance as well as resistance to their own effect (unpublished observations). Auto-induction of resistance to TNF could not be related to depletion of receptors to the protein. As shown in Fig. 9, within a few hours of removal of TNF, which had been applied to the cell at saturating concentrations, free cell-surface receptors for the protein were replenished, yet the extent of resistance to TNF cytotoxicity induced by such pretreatment remained unchanged. It therefore seems likely that this resistance indeed reflects the activation by TNF of mechanisms that counteract its cytotoxic effects.

Recently we have noticed that, besides TNF and LT, several other cytokines, including insulin and interleukin-1 (IL-1) can induce in cells resistance to the cytotoxicity of the CTXs. Further examination of the protective effect of IL-1 revealed induction, by this cytokine, of a rapid and effective decrease in cell surface receptors to TNF. That decrease could not fully account for the protective effect of IL-1 since following the removal of IL-1 TNF receptors were rapidly replenished yet the cells remained resistant to the cytotoxicity of TNF (Holtmann, Hahn and Wallach, submitted).

The potentiation of CTX effects by IFN can be related in part to an IFN-induced increase in the number of CTX receptors. As shown in Table IV, cells of several lines show an increase in binding of ^{125}I-TNF following treatment with IFN-γ. Some of these cells also display such an increase when treated by IFN-α. An IFN-induced increase in binding of TNF has also been recently observed by others (Tsujimoto *et al.*, 1986; Aggarwal *et al.*, 1985b and Ruggiero *et al.*, 1986). These studies indicate that this IFN effect reflects an increase in amounts of the receptor protein, apparently as a consequence of its increased synthesis. It is unlikely, though, that this moderate IFN-induced increase in receptor density fully accounts for the pronounced potentiation of CTX function by IFN (compare the increase in receptor level to cytotoxic effect in Fig. 10). Other IFN-induced changes are probably also involved. Perhaps the increased sensitivity of IFN-treated cells to the cytotoxic effect of CTXs reflects not only potentiation of the mechanisms mediating this effect but also suppression of cellular mechanisms that counteract it. Consistent with this idea, the induction of auto-resistance to

TABLE IV IFN-induced increase in receptors for TNF.

Cells	IFN (1000 U/ml)	CTX Binding (cpm/10^6 cells)	CTX Binding (relative increase)
HeLa	—	1080	1
	IFN-α	1800	1.67
	IFN-γ	2200	2.04
WISH	—	1050	1
	IFN-α	1000	0.95
	IFN-γ	1440	1.37
L-132	—	800	1
	IFN-α	1000	1.25
	IFN-γ	1040	1.3
FS11	—	440	1
	IFN-α	400	0.91
	IFN-γ	650	1.48
U937	—	920	1
	IFN-α	1300	1.41

Specific binding of radiolabelled TNF at a concentration of 2 U/ml (U937 cells) and 10 U/ml (other cells) was determined following 12 hours treatment by rIFN-α or rIFN-γ at 1000 U/ml. (Israel *et al.*, 1985).

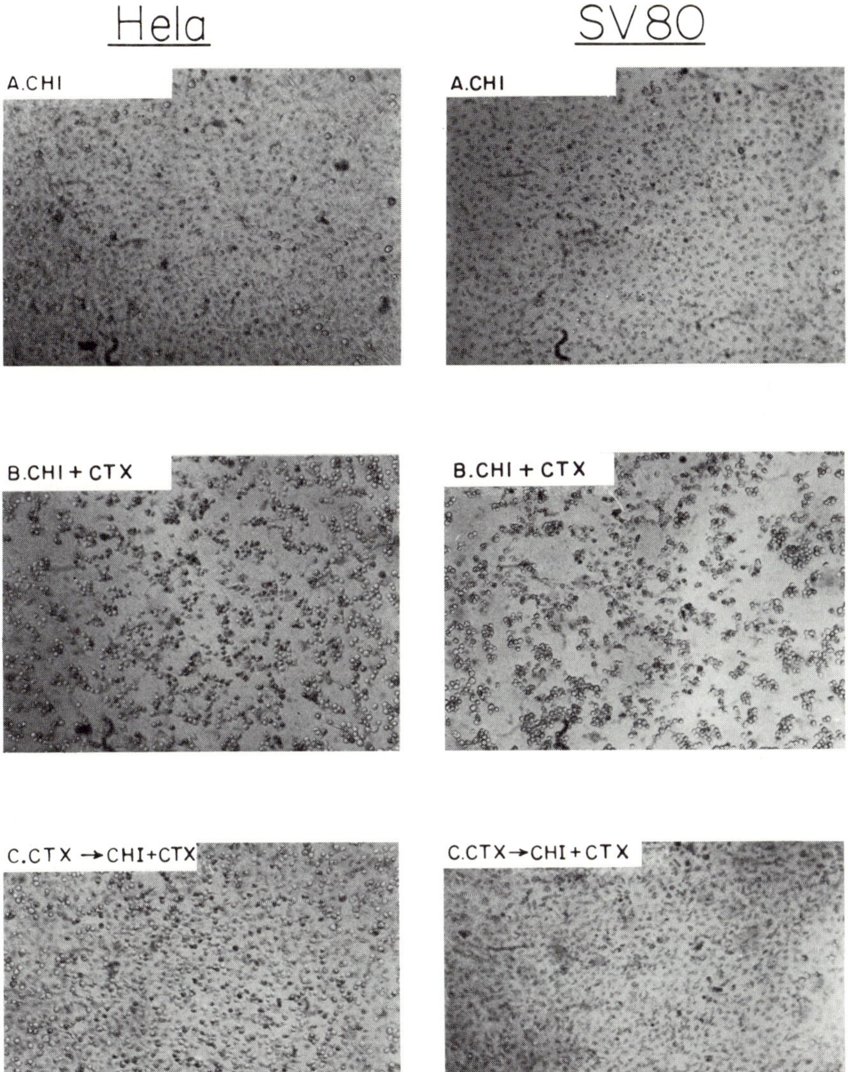

Fig. 8 Auto-induction of resistance to the cytotoxic effect of CTXs. The killing of HeLa and SV80 cells by a crude preparation of PHA-induced human CTXs (8 U/ml), incubated for 12 hours together with CHI (50 μg/ml) (B), compared with the normal morphology of the cells observed on incubation with CHI alone (A). The extent of killing is markedly reduced in cells which were pretreated for 3 hours with CTXs (80 U/ml) in the absence of CHI, rinsed and treated again with CTX (8 U/ml) this time in the presence of CHI (C) (Wallach, 1984).

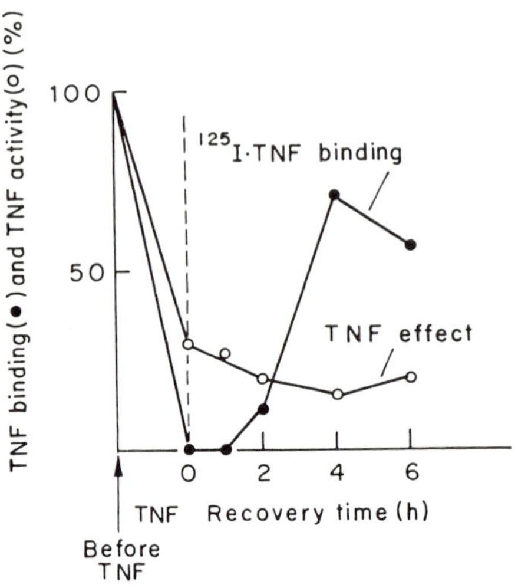

Fig. 9 Lack of correlation between TNF receptor concentration and decrease in vulnerability to its cytotoxic effect following pretreatment of L132 human cells with TNF. L132 human cells were incubated for 2 hours with TNF (260 U/ml), rinsed and further incubated in TNF-free medium. At various times the ability of the cells to bind TNF and to respond to its cytotoxic effect was measured; the former by binding of ^{125}I-labelled TNF (60 U/ml) and the latter by measuring the cytotoxicity of TNF (7 U/ml) in the presence of CHI. Results are presented at per cent of TNF bound specificially (960 c.p.m./10^5 cells) and of the cytotoxic titre of the test sample of TNF, observed before pretreatment by TNF (Israel *et al.*, 1986).

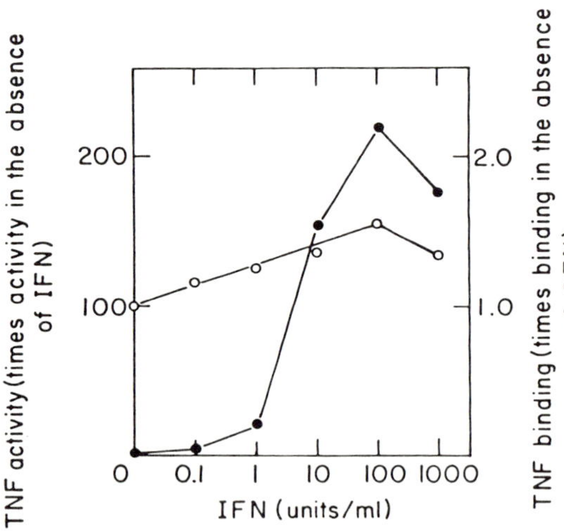

Fig. 10 Titration of the effect of IFN-γ on the cytotoxic activity of human TNF (solid symbols) and on the binding of the protein to its receptors (open symbols) in human HeLa cells. Cells were incubated for 12 hours with the indicated concentrations of IFN-γ. Their vulnerability to the cytotoxic effect of TNF was then determined by titrating; in the presence of CHI, the cytotoxic activity of a given preparation of TNF (titre of 530 U/ml in cells not treated by IFN). Binding of TNF was determined by incubating the cells with saturating levels of ^{125}I-TNF (7500 U/ml). In cells not treated by IFN, specific binding of 1000 c.p.m./10^5 cells was observed (Israel *et al.*, 1986).

TNF, described above, is found to be greatly reduced in cells treated by IFN (unpublished results).

V ON THE PHYSIOLOGICAL ROLE OF THE CTXs

There is little information available on the formation and function *in vivo* of CTXs. The physiological role of these proteins can, therefore, only be a matter of speculation, on the basis of our present fragmentary knowledge of the way these proteins are formed and function *in vitro*. The following implications of that knowledge seem to me particularly worthy of emphasis.

(1) It seems reasonable to assume that the CTXs function against their inducing agents; these are found to be quite heterogeneous. Thus, a bacterial product (LPS), a virus (Sendai virus), a T cell mitogenic agent (PHA), and tumour cells have all been found to induce TNF. Like the IFNs, CTXs may, therefore, play a rather non-specific role in the immune response, contributing to the defence against a variety of pathogenic agents. Indeed, one may infer a heterogeneity of functions for CTXs from the way they affect cells: a role for TNF in the immune response to viral infection may be indicated by the increased vulnerability to its cytotoxic effect in cells infected by certain viruses. An antibacterial role is perhaps indicated by the augmentation of phagocytic activity of granulocytes by TNF and an anti-tumour role by its cytotoxic effect against certain tumour cell lines.

(2) Some of the leukocyte-mediated cytotoxic activities (such as that of the cytotoxic T lymphocytes) are found to be exerted solely against those target cells to which these leukocytes bind. Involvement of CTXs in such "contact-dependent" cytotoxic activities has often been suggested, but remains to be confirmed. Even if it turns out that TNF or LT do take part, it is unlikely to be their sole function. The fact that those proteins can be induced by both cellular and non-cellular inducers (such as LPS) and the way the CTXs function, by binding avidly to cell surface receptors, which should allow them to affect remote target cells, strongly suggest that TNF and LT have a role as mediators which function distantly from their producing cells.

(3) We might understand the function of CTXs better if we bear in mind that these proteins are likely to be produced in areas of inflammation; specifically in inflammation reflected in delayed-type hypersensitivity (DTH). Indeed, among the T lymphocytes, the ones believed to be most involved in DTH (the Lyt 1^+ cells) are those found to produce the CTXs (Eardley *et al.*, 1980; Tite *et al.*, 1985). In the micro-environment formed by "walling off" the inflammatory area as a result of lymphatic blockage, CTXs may function more effectively. They may reach a high concentration

along with IFNs produced *in situ* which can potentiate the actions of the CTXs. The cytotoxic functions of the CTXs, found to be greatly increased at elevated temperatures *in vitro* (Peter *et al.*, 1973; Ruff and Gifford, 1981b) can be potentiated by the fever in the area of inflammation. Limited supply of nutrients and of oxygen to this region may sensitize cells to the cytotoxic effect of CTXs, similarly to the sensitization observed *in vitro* when applying metabolic blockers to cells. Accumulation of MP and of granulocytes at the site of delayed type hypersensitivity, where CTXs are likely to be formed, should allow these cells to respond to the immunoregulatory effects of the CTXs. In addition, response of remote tissues to the CTXs leaking into the circulation from the site of inflammation, such as the inhibition of lipoprotein-lipase by TNF, may contribute to the defence at the level of the whole organism. Unfortunately, most information on the role of DTH reactions relates to the pathological implications of this inflammatory response (tissue damage caused in viral infection, graft rejection, etc.). This information may provide clues to the nature of situations in which CTX formation is deleterious, but gives little idea of what positive functions the CTXs can fulfil.

(4) Although the function of CTXs is not antigen-specific, there does appear to be some selectivity in their effects. That selectivity is dictated firstly by dependence of the function of CTXs (at least the function of TNF and LT) on cell surface receptors to those proteins. While the amounts of these receptors are known to vary, there is no information yet on the physiological parameters that control the variation, other than the fact that some increase in the receptor level can be induced by IFN. (As mentioned above (see page 113) we have recently noted that TNF receptors are subjected also to effective modulation by interleukin-1. Unlike the IFN-induced increase in TNF receptors which appears to reflect increased synthesis of the receptor protein, the IL-1 induced decrease in receptors for TNF is independent of protein synthesis, and probably reflects uptake or inactivation of the receptors (Holtmann and Wallach, submitted).) Further selectivity may be imposed on the function of CTXs by the dependence of their cytotoxic effect on a prior sensitization of the affected cell. Although the biochemical nature of the sensitization mechanism is not known, it appears, by the nature of those agents known to sensitize cells (metabolic blockers, viruses and x-radiation), that it is due to interference with some vital functions of the cell. CTXs can thus be viewed as agents with the capacity for distinguishing between "healthy" cells, which can resist their cytotoxicity and thus be spared from killing, and "sick" cells, which fail to resist CTX cytotoxicity and are therefore specifically eliminated.

(5) At present, there is no solid evidence for a specific anti-tumour role of CTXs, linking vulnerability of the tumour cell to CTXs with a specific

characteristic of malignancy—for example, the growth of the cells independently of supply of growth-factors or the activation of specific oncogenes. Yet the mere fact that some kinds of tumour cells respond to the cytotoxic or cytostatic effects of CTXs, even though they have failed to respond to mechanisms that normally restrain cell growth, is potentially applicable in tumour therapy (see Rundell and Evans, 1981; Ruff and Gifford, 1981a; Lee *et al.*, 1984). Perhaps it will be possible to direct CTX activity selectively against tumour cells, taking advantage of the fact that DNA-intercalating drugs and ionizing radiation, which preferentially affect rapidly-growing tumour cells, sensitize cells to the cytotoxic effect of CTXs. From the point of view of IFN research, the most intriguing question is whether effects of CTXs on tumour cells and their synergism with IFN can contribute to increasing the effectiveness of IFN in tumour therapy: do CTXs produced *in situ*, formed in increased amounts owing to the enhancement of CTX formation by IFN, contribute to some of the anti-tumour effects that IFNs have already been found to exert, and can CTXs, injected into patients together with IFN, further potentiate these anti-tumour effects?

VI CONCLUDING REMARKS

While there is some recent information on the structure of CTXs, our knowledge of their function, the mechanisms involved, and their physiological role is still quite limited. Basically what has been learned in the short time that purified CTXs have been available is that the way in which CTXs function is more complex than was believed hitherto. The cytotoxic activity of the CTXs had been thought to be non-specific, leading to killing of "innocent bystander cells". A more thorough examination now shows that this activity can be subjected to effective modulation, depending on the nature of the target cell and its metabolic state. Furthermore, when they do not exert cytotoxic effects, CTXs mediate other regulatory functions.

Which of the various effects of CTX function observed *in vitro* leads to physiologically meaningful consequences is not known. Nor can we tell yet whether the practical benefits of these proteins, such as the killing of tumour cells synergistically with IFN, will be found sufficiently effective to be applicable in therapy. Perhaps it will be the adverse effects, such as mediation of cachexia or of shock symptoms in disease, that will turn out to be the more prominent, necessitating a search for means of suppressing CTX activity. We know that TNF and LT do not act simply by exerting an enzymatic activity but rather by binding to specific receptors, thus activating cellular mechanisms that affect gene regulation and can also mediate cell death. The nature of those mechanisms is yet to be elucidated. Knowledge of the mechanisms initiating synthesis of CTXs within the CTX-producing cells is also quite limited.

Our present incomplete state of knowledge of the CTXs provides intriguing hints toward a deeper understanding in the future. The lack of resemblance between the TNFs (TNF and LT) and other known proteins; the way these proteins kill cells; the presence of receptors to TNF and LT on many differing cells; the ability of TNF and LT to initiate cellular responses other than cell death; and the multiplicity of agents that induce production of these proteins, all indicate that further studies on these proteins, as well as of the way their formation and function are regulated by IFN, may disclose novel information on mechanisms controlling the life and death of cells and on ways whereby the immune response can regulate these mechanisms.

ACKNOWLEDGEMENTS

I gratefully acknowledge the many colleagues who provided me with published and unpublished material for this review. I wish also to thank Professor Michel Revel for helpful discussions and Professor Joseph Korn, Professor Edward Simon, Dr Dan Aderka and Mrs Myra Kay for their comments on the manuscript.

Research in the author's laboratory was supported by grants from the National Council of Research and Development (Israel), Inter-Yeda Ltd, the Leukemia Research Foundation (Chicago), and from the Fund for Basic Research, administered by the Israel Academy for Science and Humanities.

REFERENCES

Adams, D. O. (1980). *J. Immunol.* **124**, 286–292.

Aderka, D., Novick, D., Hahn, T., Fischer, D. G. and Wallach, D. (1985). *Cell Immunol.* **92**, 218–225.

Aderka, D., Holtmann, H., Toker, L., Hahn, T. and Wallach, D. (1986a) *J. Immunol.* **136**, 2938–2942.

Aderka, D., Levo, Y., Ramot, B., Michalevicz, R., Meytes, D., Shaklai, M., Hahn, T., Holtmann, H., Revel, M. and Wallach, D. (1986b). (submitted).

Adolf, G. R. (1984). An abstract presented in the fourth International Lymphokine Workshop, p. 231.

Aggarwal, B. B., Moffat, B. and Harkins, N. R. (1984). *J. Biol. Chem.* **259**, 686–691.

Aggarwal, B. B., Kohr, W. J., Hass, P. E., Moffat, B., Spencer, S. A., Henzel, W. J., Bringman, T. S., Nedwin, G. E., Goeddel, D. V. and Harkins, R. N. (1985). *J. Biol. Chem.* **260**, 2345–2354.

Basham, T. X. and Merigan, T. S. (1983). *J. Immunol.* **130**, 1492–1495.

Bertolini, D. R., Nedwin, G. E., Bringman, T. S., Smith, D. D. and Mundy, G. R. (1986). *Nature* (*London*) **319**, 516–518.

Beutler, B., Greenwald, D., Hulmes, J. D., Chang, M., Pan, E. Y-C., Mathison, J., Ulevitch, R., and Cerami, A. (1985a). *Nature* (*London*) **316**, 552–554.

Beutler, B., Milsark, I. W. and Cerami, A. C. (1985b). *Science* **229**, 869–871.

Beutler, B. A. and Cerami, A. (1985c). *J. Immunol.* **135**, 3963–3971.

Carswell, E. A., Old, L. J., Kassel, R. L., Green, S., Fiore, N. and Williamson, B. (1975). *Proc. Natl Acad. Sci. USA* **72**, 3666–3670.

Chang, E. H., Mims, S. J., Trich, T. J. and Friedman, R. M. (1977). *J. Gen. Virol.* **34**, 363–367.

Chang, R. and Lee, S. H. (1985). An abstract presented in the 1985 TNO meeting on the Interferon System, p. 55.

Chroboczek-Kelker, H., Oppenheim, J. D., Stone-Wolff, D., Henriksen-De Stefano, D., Aggarwal, B. B., Stevenson, H. C. and Vilček, J. (1985). *Int. J. Cancer.* **36**, 69–73.

Collins, T., Lapierre, L. A., Fiers, W., Strominger, J. L. and Pober, J. S. (1986). *Proc. Natl Acad. Sci. USA* **83**, 446–450.

Content, J., De Wit, L., Poupart, P., Opdenakker, G., Van-Damme, J. and Billiau, J. (1985). *Eur. J. Biochem.* **152**, 253–257.

Currie, G. A. (1978). *Nature* (*London*) **273**, 758–759.

Darzynkiewicz, Z., Williamson, B., Carswell, E. A. and Old, L. J. (1984). *Cancer Res.* **44**, 83–90.

Dayer, J.-M., Zavadil-Grob, C., Ucla, C. and Mach, B. (1984). *Eur. J. Immunol.* **14**, 898–901.

Dayer, J-M., Beutler, B. and Cerami, A. (1985). *J. Exp. Med.* **162**, 2163–2168.

Dewhirst, F. E., Stashenko, P. P., Mole, J. E. and Tsurumachi, T. (1985). *J. Immunol.* **135**, 2562–2568.

Eardley, D. D., Shen, F. W., Gershon, R. K. and Ruddle, N. H. (1980). *J. Immunol.* **124**, 1199–1202.

Eifel, P., Billingsley, A. and Lucas, J. Z. (1979). *Cell. Immunol.* **47**, 197–203.

Farram, E. and Targan, S. R. (1983) *J. Immunol.* **130**, 1252–1256.

Fiers, W., Brouckaert, P., Guisez, Y., Remaut, E., Varn Roy F., Devos, R., Fransen, L., Leroux, R.-G., Marmenout, A., Tavernier, J. and Van der Heyden, J. (1986). *In* "The Biology of the Interferon System". Elsevier, Amsterdam (in press).

Fransen, L., Müller, R., Marmenout, A., Tavernier, J., Van der Heyden, J., Kawashima, E., Chollet, A., Tizard, R., Van-Heuverswyn, H., Van Vliet, A., Ruyscchaert, M-R. and Fiers, W. (1985). *Nucleic Acids Res.* **13**, 4417–4429.

Gamble, J. R., Harlan, J. M., Klebanoff, S. J. and Vadas, M. A. (1985). *Proc. Natl Acad. Sci. USA* **82**, 8667–8671.

Gifford, G. E., Fick, D. A., Abd Allah, N. A. and Fisch, H. (1984). *J. Natl Cancer Inst.* **73**, 69–73.

Granger, G. A. and Kolb, W. P. (1968). *J. Immunol.* **101**, 111–120.

Granger, G. A., Yamamoto, R. S., Fair, D. S. and Hiserodt, J. C. (1978). *Cell. Immunol.* **38**, 388–402.

Gray, W. P., Aggarwal, B. B., Benton, C. V., Bringman, T. S., Henzel, W. J., Jarret, J. A., Leung, D. W., Moffat, B., Sverdersky, Ng L. P., Palladino, M. A. Jr. and Nedwin, G. E. (1984). *Nature* (*London*) **312**, 721–724.

Hahn, T., Toker, L., Budilovsky, S., Aderka, D., Eshhar, Z. and Wallach, D. (1985). *Proc. Natl Acad. Sci. USA* **82**, 3814–3818.

Haranaka, K., Satomi, N., Sakurai, A. and Nariuchi, H. (1985). *Int. J. Cancer* **36**, 395–400.

Hass, P. E., Hotchkiss, A., Mohler, M. and Aggarwal, B. B. (1985). *J. Biol. Chem.* **260**, 12214–12218.

Hiserodt, J. C., Ware, C. F., Harris, P. C. and Granger, G. A. (1977). *Cell Immunol.* **34**, 326–339.

Hiserodt, J. C., Ford, S. C., Harris, P. C. and Granger, G. A. (1979). *Cell. Immunol.* **47**, 32–45.

Israel, S., Hahn, T., Holtmann, H. and Wallach, D. (1986). *Immunol. letters.* **12**, 217–227.

Kildahl-Andersen, O., Espevik, T. and Nissen-Meyer, J. (1985). *Cell. Immunol.* **95**, 392–406.

Klostergaard, J., Yamamoto, R. S. and Granger, G. A. (1981). *In* "Lymphokines and Thymic Hormones: their Potential Utilization in Cancer Therapeutics" (A. L. Goldstein and M. A. Chirigios, eds.), pp. 95–108. Raven Press, New York.

Kohase, M. Henrikson-De Stefano, D., May, L. T., Vilček, J. and Sehgal, P. B. (1986). *Cell* (in press).

Knop, J., Stremmer, R., Neumann, C., De Maeyer, E. J. and Macher, E. (1982). *Nature* (*London*) **296**, 717–719.

Kull, F. C. and Cuatrecasas, P. (1985). *Proc. Natl Acad. Sci. USA* **81**, 7932–7936.

Kull, F. C., Jacobs, S. and Cuatrecasas, P. (1985) *Proc. Natl Acad. Sci. USA* **82**, 5756–5760.

Lee, S. H., Aggarwal, B. B., Rinderknecht, E., Assisi, F. and Chiu, H. (1984). *J. Immunol.* **133**, 1083–1086.

Lindahl, P., Leary, P. and Gresser, I. (1974). *Eur. J. Immunol.* **4**, 779–794.

Männel, D. N., Moore, R. N. and Mergenhagen, S. E. (1980). *Infect. Immunol.* **30**, 523–530.

Männel, D. N., Falk, W. and Meltzer, M. S. (1981). *Infect. Immunol.* **33**, 156–164.

Marmenout, A., Fransen, L., Tavernier, J., Van Der Heyden, J., Tizard, R., Kawashima, E., Shaw, A., Johnson, M-J., Semon, D., Muller, R., Ruysschaert, M-R., Van Vliet, A. and Fiers, W. (1985). *Eur. J. Biochem.* **152**, 515–522.

Matthews, N. (1979). *Br. J. Cancer* **40**, 534–539.

Metcalf, D. (1975). *In* "A Training Manual For Cancer Research Workers", (ed. D. Metcalf). UICC Technical Report Series, Vol. 20, p. 177.

Menkin, V. (1943). *Science* **97**, 165–168.

Nedwin, G. E., Sverdersky, L. P., Bringman, T. S., Palladino, M. A. Jr. and Goeddel, D. V. (1985). *J. Immunol.* **135**, 2492–2497.

Onozaki, K., Matsushima, K., Aggarwal, B. B. and Oppenheim, J. J. (1985). *J. Immunol.* **135**, 3962–3968.

Ortaldo, J. R., Palladino, M., Sayers, T., Denn, A. C. III., Shephard, M. and Herberman, R. B. (1985). An abstract presented in the 7th European Immunology Meeting, p. 91.

Ostrove, J. N. and Gifford, G. E. (1979). *Proc. Soc. Exp. Biol. Med.* **160**, 354–358.

Pauker, K., Cantell, K. and Henle, W. (1962). *Virology* **17**, 324–334.

Pennica, D., Nedwin, G. E., Hayflick, J. S., Seeburg, P. W., Derynck, R., Pallidino, M. A., Kohr, W. J., Aggarwal, B. B. and Goeddel, D. V. (1984). *Nature* (*London*) **312**, 724–729.

Pennica, D., Hayflick, J. S., Bringman, T. S., Palladino, M. A. and Goeddel, D. V. (1985). *Proc. Natl Acad. Sci. USA* **82**, 6060–6064.

Peter, J. B., Stratton, J. A., Stempel, K. E., Yu, D. and Cardin, C. (1973). *J. Immunol.* **111**, 770–782.

Pincus, W. B. (1967). *J. Reticuloendotheliol. Soc.* **4**, 122–139.

Pober, J. S., Bevilacqua, M. P., Mendrick, D. L., Lapierre, L. A., Fiers, W. and Grimbrane, M. A. Jr. (1986) *J. Immunol.* **136**, 1680–1687.

Podak, E. R. (1985). *Immunol. Today* **6**, 21–27.
Ransom, J. H., Evans, C. H., McCabe, R. P., Pomato, N., Heinbaugh, J. A., Chin, M. and Hanna, M. G. (1985). *Cancer Res.* **45**, 851–862.
Roberts, A. B., Anzano, M. A., Wakefield, L. M., Roche, N. S., Stern, D. F. and Sporn, M. B. (1985). *Proc. Natl Acad. Sci. USA* **82**, 119–123.
Rosenau, W. (1980). *Int. J. Immunopharmacol.* **3**, 1–8.
Rosenau, W., Goldberg, M. L. and Burke, G. C. (1973). *J. Immunol.* **111**, 1128–1135.
Rubin, B. V., Anderson, S. L., Sullivan, S. A., Williamson, B. D., Carswell, E. A. and Old, L. J. (1985). *Proc. Natl Acad. Sci. USA* **82**, 6637–6641.
Ruddle, N. H. and Waksman, B. H. (1968). *J. Exp. Med.* **128**, 1267–1279.
Ruddle, N. H., Powell, M. B. and Conta, B. S. (1983). *Lymphokine Res.* **2**, 23–30.
Ruff, M. R. and Gifford, G. E. (1981a). *In* "Lymphokines", (E. Pick and M. Landy, eds.), pp. 235–272. Academic Press, New York.
Ruff, M. R. and Gifford, G. E. (1981b). *Infect. Immunol.* **31**, 380–385.
Ruggiero, V., Tavernier, J., Fiers, W. and Baglioni, C. (1986). *J. Immunol.* **136**, 2445–2450.
Rundell, J. O. and Evans, C. H. (1981). *Immunopharmacology* **3**, 9–18.
Schleimer, R. P. and Rutledge, B. K. (1986). *J. Immunol.* **136**, 649–654.
Schmidt, J. A., Mizel, S. B., Cohen, D. and Green, I. (1982). *J. Immunol.* **128**, 2177–2182.
Shalaby, M. R., Aggarwal, B. B., Rinderknecht, E., Svedersky, L. P., Finkle, B. S. and Palladino, M. A. Jr. (1985a). *J. Immunol.* **135**, 2069–2073.
Shalaby, M. R., Hirabayashi, S. E., Svedersky, L. P. and Palladino, M. A. Jr. (1985b). *Fed. Proc.* **44**, 569.
Shirai, T., Yamaguchi, H., Ito, H., Tudd, C. W. and Wallace, R. B. (1985). *Nature* (*London*) **313**, 803–806.
Steinhauer, E. H., Doyle, A. T. and Kadish, A. S. (1985). *J. Immunol.* **135**, 294–299.
Stone-Wolff, D. S., Yip, Y. K., Chroboczek-Kelker, H., Le, J., Henriksen-DeStefano, D., Rubin, B. Y., Rinderknecht, E., Aggarwal, B. B. and Vilček, J. (1984). *J. Exp. Med.* **159**, 828–843.
Sugarman, B. J., Aggarwal, B. B., Hass, P. E., Figari, I. S., Palladino, M. A. Jr. and Shephard, H. M. (1985). *Science* **230**, 943–945.
Sverdersky, L. P., Nedwin, G. E., Bringman, T. S., Shalaby, M., Lamott, J. A., Goeddel, D. V. and Palladino, M. A. Jr. (1985a). *Fed. Proc.* **44**, 589.
Sverdersky, L. P., Nedwin, G. E., Goeddel, D. V. and Palladino, M. A. Jr. (1985b). *J. Immunol.* **134**, 1604–1608.
Tite, J. P., Powell, M. B. and Ruddle, N. H. (1985). *J. Immunol.* **135**, 25–33.
Torti, F. M., Dieckmann, B., Beutler, B., Cerami, A. and Ringold, G. M. (1985). *Science* **229**, 867–869.
Trinchieri, G. and Santoli, D. (1978). *J. Exp. Med.* **147**, 1314–1333.
Tsujimoto, M., Yip, Y. K. and Vilček, J. (1985). *Proc. Natl Acad. Sci. USA* **82**, 7626–7630.
Tsujimoto, M., Yip, Y. K. and Vilček, J. (1986). *J. Immunol.* **136**, 2441–2444.
Vilček, J., Henriksen-DeStefano, D., Palombella, V. J. and Tsujimoto, M. (1986). *In* "The Biology of the Interferon System". Elsevier, Amsterdam, (in press).
Wallach, D., Fellous, M. and Revel, M. (1982). *Nature* (*London*) **299**, 833–836.
Wallach, D. (1983). *Cell. Immunol.* **75**, 390–395.
Wallach, D. and Hahn, T. (1983). *Cell. Immunol.* **76**, 390–396.
Wallach, D., Aderka, D., Budilovsky, S. and Hahn, T. (1983). *In* "The Biology of the Interferon System" (E. Demaeyer and H. Schellekens eds.), pp. 293–303, Elsevier, Amsterdam.

Wallach, D. (1984). *J. Immunol.* **132**, 2464–2469.
Wallach, D., Hahn, T. and Budilovsky, S. (1984). *FEBS Lett.* **178**, 257–263.
Wang, A. M., Creasey, A. A., Ladner, M. B., Lin, L. S., Strickler, J., Van Arodell, J. N., Yamamoto, R. and Mark, D. F. (1985). *Science* **228**, 149–154.
Ware, C. F. and Granger, G. A. (1979). *J. Immunol.* **122**, 1763–1770.
Williams, T. W. and Granger, G. A. (1973). *Cell. Immunol.* **6**, 171–185.
Williams, T. W. and Bellanti, J. A. (1983). *J. Immunol.* **130**, 518–520.
Williamson, R. D., Carswell, E. A., Rubin, B. Y., Prendergast, J. S. and Old, L. J. (1983). *Proc. Natl Acad. Sci. USA* **80**, 5397–5401.
Wong, G. and Goeddel, D. (1985). An abstract presented in the 1985 TNO meeting on the Interferon System.
Wright, S. C. and Bonavida, B. (1982). *J. Immunol.* **129**, 433–439.
Wright, S. C. and Bonavida, B. (1983a). *J. Immunol.* **130**, 2960–2964.
Wright, S. C. and Bonavida, B. (1983b). *J. Immunol.* **130**, 2965–2968.
Young, Y. D-E., Hengarter, H., Podack, E. R. and Cohn, Z. A. (1986). *Cell* **44**, 843–859.

Peroxide and Pteridine: A Hypothesis on the Regulation of Macrophage Antimicrobial Activity by Interferon γ

CARL F. NATHAN

*Laboratory of Cellular Physiology and Immunology, The Rockefeller University, New York, NY 10021 USA.**

I INTRODUCTION

Actions of interferon gamma (IFN-γ) on cells of the immune system are so pleiotypic that it can be difficult to put them in perspective. Which are physiological, which artefact? Which are critical, which incidental? When they conflict, which predominate? Beyond the task of sorting out these functions lies a challenge of another kind, posed by actions of IFN-γ for which no role has been proposed. Such puzzles hint at facets of IFN-γ yet unforeseen.

Consider neopterin, a pteridine secreted in abundance by human macrophages only after they have been exposed to IFN-γ. Picomolar concentrations of IFN-γ induce its secretion *in vitro*, and IFN-γ is one of the few cytokines among many tested that stimulate its release. A variety of other cell types, when exposed to IFN-γ, secrete no neopterin. Neopterin plays no known role in mammalian physiology. Its precursor can give rise to

**Present address: Division of Hematology-Oncology, Department of Medicine, Cornell University Medical College, 1300 York Avenue, New York, NY 10021, USA.*

INTERFERON 7
ISBN 0 12 302256 8

biopterin, a cofactor in neurotransmitter synthesis, but macrophages do not seem to make biopterin. Neopterin itself is an intermediate in a biosynthetic path whose final product, folic acid, is made by many microorganisms but not animals—a path energetically costly to traverse. Why would evolution permit a truncated and presumably vestigial form of such a path to be retained? Why assign it to the macrophage, and why make it highly inducible by IFN-γ?

In contrast to the mystery surrounding neopterin is the regulation by IFN-γ of oxidative metabolism in macrophages, leading to enhanced capacity to secrete incompletely reduced forms of molecular oxygen, such as superoxide and hydrogen peroxide. Present evidence leaves little doubt that the latter response plays a major (but not exclusive) role in the antimicrobial capacity of immunologically activated macrophages, a capacity itself inducible by IFN-γ. This fits readily into the premise that the chief physiological role of the interferons is to combat infection. Indeed, it supports the view that the main function of IFN-α and IFN-β may be to induce antiviral activity in most host cells, while IFN-γ may be specialized to induce antibacterial, antiprotozoal and antifungal activity in those cells likely to harbor such pathogens. In addition to macrophages (Edward *et al.*, 1985; Horwitz, 1985; Kiderlen *et al.*, 1984; McCabe *et al.*, 1984; Murray *et al.*, 1983a, 1985; Nathan *et al*, 1983a; Ockenhouse *et al.*, 1984; Peck, 1985; Plata *et al.*, 1984; Rothermel *et al.*, 1983; Schreiber *et al.*, 1985; Wirth *et al.*, 1985; Wisseman and Waddell, 1983; Wu-Hsieh *et al.*, 1984), such cells may include endothelium (Wisseman and Waddell, 1983), fibroblasts (Byrne and Krueger, 1983; Pfefferkorn, 1984; Plata *et al.*, 1984; Wisseman and Waddell 1983), and certain parenchymal cells, such as hepatocytes in malaria and Q fever.

I will first review the evidence for IFN-γ's regulation of each of these two macrophage secretory products, peroxide and pteridine. I will then speculate on their possible commonality of function, with a hypothesis that relates neopterin secretion to the view that the chief physiological function of IFN-γ may be the induction in host cells of antibacterial, antiprotozoal and antifungal states.

II REGULATION OF THE MACROPHAGE RESPIRATORY BURST BY IFN-γ

The following discussion uses the term "macrophage activation" to refer to enhanced capacity of macrophages to inhibit intracellular microbial pathogens, and considers an enhanced capacity of the macrophage to secrete reactive oxygen intermediates as a biochemical marker of the activated state. The evidence that reactive oxygen intermediates play a major role in

TABLE I Evidence for Involvement of Reactive Oxygen Intermediates (ROI) in Macrophage Antimicrobial Activity[a]

I. Correlations
   (a) Between the antimicrobial activity of a given macrophage population and its capacity to secrete ROI when suitably triggered.
   (b) Between the susceptibility of a pathogen to killing by macrophages and its ability to trigger the production of ROI.
   (c) Between the resistance of a pathogen to killing by macrophages and its resistance to killing by ROI.
   (d) Between the resistance of a pathogen to killing by macrophages and the specific activity or content of its antioxidant defences.

II. Interventions
   (a) Inhibition of killing of a pathogen by interventions designed to decrease the level of ROI within macrophages.
   (b) Enhancement of killing of a pathogen by interventions designed to raise the level of ROI within macrophages
   (c) Enhancement of killing of a pathogen by interventions designed to augment the cytotoxic potential of a given level of ROI.

[a] Adapted from Nathan (1983b).

macrophage antimicrobial defense derives largely from experiments with *Trypanosoma cruzi, Toxoplasma gondii, Leishmania* spp., *Candida* spp., *Mycobacterium microti,* and *Plasmodium falciparum.* The experiments supporting this conclusion are categorized in Table I, adapted from Nathan (1983b), where the details are reviewed.

In the mid 1960s, Mackaness established that macrophage activation is immunologically inducible and that its agent is the antigen-triggered lymphocyte (Mackaness, 1970). By the early 1970s, it was apparent that the activating signal from lymphocytes was delivered via soluble, secreted glycoproteins (Nathan *et al.*, 1971, 1973; Fowles *et al.*, 1973), operationally called macrophage activating factors or MAFs. Purification and identification of MAFs was frustrated for years by their extremely low concentration in biologically active preparations and by the difficulty of their bioassay. Within the last three years, there has been rapid progress, thanks to the application of monoclonal antibodies, improvement of chromatographic systems, and production of proteins from cloned, recombinant genes. This recent evidence indicates that for the protozoal and bacterial pathogens studied, IFN-γ is the predominant MAF produced by clonally unselected lymphocytes, although there seem to be other MAFs demonstrable in the media of certain lymphoid clones.

Five lines of evidence support the identification of IFN-γ as the predominant lymphocyte-derived MAF in the sense defined above. Three of

TABLE II Evidence that the Lymphokine Enhancing Human Macrophage Oxidative Metabolism is IFN-γ[a]

Lymphokine preparation and means of induction	Concentration before dilution, or specific activity	Macrophage H_2O_2 release: Ratio, exp[b] over control	Macrophage H_2O_2 release: % Inhibition by anti-IFN-γ mAb
Crude lymphokines			
lentil lectin + mez.[c]	1–10 × 10^2 U/ml	3.8 ± 1.5 (6)	207[d] ± 43 (3)
concanavalin A	1–3 × 10^3 U/ml	3.6 ± 0.5 (5)	86 ± 9 (5)
toxoplasma antigen	2–6 × 10^3 U/ml	4.1 ± 0.5 (4)	108 ± 12 (4)
Purified native IFN-γ			
lentil lectin + mez.	10^6 U/mg	7.2 ± 1.9 (4)	113 ± 8 (2)
staph. enterotoxin A	10^7 U/mg	9.7 ± 2.4 (8)	91 ± 13 (5)
Recombinant IFN-γ	3 × 10^6 U/mg	17.7 ± 4.8 (14)	

[a] Data from Nathan *et al.* (1983a). Table reprinted from Nathan and Tsunawaki (1986).

[b] Exp = experimental. Mean ± SEM for 41 experimental sets = 643 ± 57 nmol H_2O_2/mg cell protein/hour.

[c] mez. = mezerein.

[d] Inhibition > 100% represents unmasking of suppressive activity in the mezerein-induced supernate.

these are summarized in Table II. First, human peripheral blood lymphocytes stimulated with any of three different polyclonal or oligoclonal activators, including both mitogens and antigen, secreted IFN-γ. The IFN-γ-containing, lymphocyte-conditioned media quadrupled the ability of human macrophages, derived by culture of blood monocytes, to secrete H_2O_2 when challenged with phorbol myristate acetate. The enhancing effect was abolished by incubating the lymphokines with a monoclonal antibody that neutralizes IFN-γ. This suggested that IFN-γ was necessary for macrophage activation by these supernatants, but did not rule out the possibility that another molecule was also required, or even that the antibody neutralized an activating factor other than IFN-γ. Second, IFN-γ was extensively (but incompletely) purified from these lymphokines by either of two independent protocols, as monitored by bioassay for antiviral activity. The active fractions were enriched in the ability to activate macrophage oxidative metabolism, virtually excluding the possibility that the monoclonal antibody fortuitously reacted with a non-IFN-γ MAF. However, it was still possible that macrophage activation required both IFN-γ and a cytokine that can co-purify extensively with IFN-γ, such as lymphotoxin (Stone-Wolff *et al.*, 1984). Third, pure, recombinant IFN-γ (rIFN-γ) was a potent macrophage

TABLE III Intracellular Nonviral Pathogens Whose Killing by Macrophages is Enhanced by IFN-γ.

Parasite	Reference
Bacteria	
Rickettsia prowazekii[a]	Wisseman and Waddell (1983)
Chlamydia psittaci	Rothermel *et al.* (1983)
Listeria monocytogenes	Peck (1985); Schreiber *et al.* (1985); Kiderlen *et al.* (1984)
Mycobacterium intracellulare	Edward (1985)
Pneumophila legionella	Horwitz (1985)
Protozoa	
Toxoplasma gondii	Nathan *et al.* (1983a)
Leishmania donovani	Murray *et al.* (1983a)
Plasmodium falciparum[b]	Ockenhouse *et al.* (1984)
Trypanosoma cruzi	Wirth *et al.* (1985), Plata *et al.* (1984)
Fungi	
Histoplasma capsulatum[c]	Wu-Hsieh *et al.* (1984)

[a] Definitive evidence that IFN-γ was the activating factor was provided in the case of fibroblasts by Turco and Winkler (1983).

[b] An intracellular parasite of erythrocytes and hepatocytes but not macrophages.

[c] Definitive identification of IFN-γ as the activating factor is still awaited.

Note added in proof: Subsequent reports have added six more pathogens to this list.

activating factor, with effective concentrations in the picomolar range (Nathan *et al.*, 1983a). The results in Table II were duplicated with regard to the ability of macrophages to kill *Toxoplasma gondii* (Nathan *et al.*, 1983a), and were confirmed for macrophage antileishmanial function (Murray *et al.*, 1983). Together, these observations support the interpretation that IFN-γ is both necessary and sufficient for macrophage activation by the lymphokine preparations studied and for the assays used.

Consistent with these observations, experiments in other laboratories have recently demonstrated IFN-γ-induced macrophage activation towards a wide range of pathogenic microorganisms. Cumulatively, these total at least ten species of bacteria, protozoa, and fungi (Table III).

However, these observations do not exclude the possibility that other cytokines may also activate macrophages, cytokines that may not have been present in sufficient concentration in the lymphocyte supernatants studied. One approach was to test individually each cytokine already known to have an effect on mononuclear phagocytes and available as highly purified and well characterized preparations (Nathan *et al.*, 1984). With rIFN-γ as a positive control in each experiment, enhanced oxidative metabolism was not observed after incubation of human macrophages with native IFN-α,

TABLE IV Comparison of IFN-γ with Other Cytokines for Induction of Antitoxoplasma Activity in Human Macrophages[a]

Agent[b]	U/ml	% Toxoplasmas killed at 4–6 hours	No. toxoplasmas/ vacuole at 20 hours
Medium	—	3.3 ± 1.6 (7)[c]	6.1 ± 0.3 (9)
rIFN-γ	100–300	42.9 ± 4.3 (7)	1.9 ± 0.1 (10)
nIFNα	300–500[d]	0.0 ± 0.0 (2)	5.2 ± 0.2 (2)
rIFNαA	300–500[d]	1.0 ± 0.7 (2)	5.8 ± 0.2 (2)
rIFNαD	300–500[d]	0.8 ± 0.7 (4)	5.1 ± 0.3 (5)
rIFNβ	300–500[d]	0.0 ± 0.0 (3)	5.0 ± 0.4 (4)
CSF-1	500	9.0 ± 4.2 (3)	5.4 ± 0.5 (3)
GM-CSF	500	2.8 ± 1.9 (4)	6.1 ± 0.3 (4)
MIF	1–30	7.2 ± 3.0 (6)	5.9 ± 0.6 (6)
nIL-2	10–100	5.0 ± 5.0 (2)	4.6 ± 0.4 (2)
rIL-2	10–100	5.5 ± 3.3 (4)	4.8 ± 0.3 (4)

[a] Reprinted from Nathan *et al.* (1984).

[b] Macrophages were incubated with the indicated cytokines for 3 days before being washed and challenged with toxoplasmas. The course of infection was followed in control medium for the next 20 hours.

[c] Mean ± SEM for the number of experiments in parentheses, each in duplicate.

[d] Higher concentrations were not tested because rounding up of the macrophages interfered with counting intracellular organisms.

rIFN-αA, rIFN-αD, rIFN-β, colony-stimulating factor type 1, colony-stimulating factor for granulocytes and macrophages, pluripotent colony-stimulating factor (an IL3-like molecule), native and recombinant interleukin-2, and native tumour necrosis factor. Recently, similar results were obtained with colony-stimulating factor (granulocyte/macrophage type) purified to homogeneity by K. Welte and E. Platzer. The reasons for discrepant results with CSF-1 in a murine system (Wing *et al.*, 1985) are not yet apparent. Migration inhibitory factor did afford some enhancement of peroxide-releasing capacity, but as shown in Table IV, this was not associated with induction of antitoxoplasma activity. These findings indicate that macrophage activation is a highly restricted property among cytokines with effects on macrophages, and provide the fourth line of evidence for the predominant role of IFN-γ in this regard.

A fifth test of the role of IFN-γ as a macrophage activating factor is whether it functions *in vivo*. Until this is demonstrated, the possibility remains that the effects observed above may be an artefact of cell culture *in vitro*. An opportunity to approach this question arose with the initiation of phase I trials of rIFN-γ in cancer patients. In order to conduct serial studies on monocytes isolated from the blood of such patients, we adapted a quantitative assay for cellular H_2O_2 production to a semi-automated microscale (de la Harpe and Nathan, 1985). Using this technique, we conducted 170 assays on cells from 13 patients with advanced malignancy who underwent 20 cycles of intravenous administration of rIFN-γ in dosages ranging from 0.1 to 1.0 mg/m^2 per infusion. Eighty-five per cent of these subjects responded by the criterion that their post-treatment monocytes released more H_2O_2 per milligram of cell protein than their pre-treatment monocytes in $\geqslant$67% of tests conducted over 1 hour after the start of infusion of rIFN-γ (Nathan *et al.*, 1985). Since monocytes can normally secrete abundant H_2O_2, they are almost surely a suboptimal population in which to look for an increase. Nonetheless, combined data for all 13 subjects revealed statistically significant increases averaging from 1.4-fold to 2.8-fold above the pre-treatment controls (Nathan *et al.*, 1985).

The above findings were perhaps the first to suggest that mononuclear phagocytes can be activated in man by a lymphocyte product. However, the physiological relevance of the demonstration is open to question, since pharmacological doses of rIFN-γ were administered to patients not known to suffer from a deficiency of endogenous IFN-γ. The hypothesis that IFN-γ may be a physiological MAF in man is being tested more stringently in patients with lepromatous leprosy (Nathan *et al.*, 1986). The dermal macrophages in such patients are packed with mycobacteria, and by this criterion are not activated, in contrast to the paucibacillary appearance of the macrophages in the tuberculoid form of the disease. Blood lymphocytes from lepromatous patients secrete little or no IFN-γ or MAF (Horwitz *et al.*, 1984) upon challenge with antigens of *M. leprae*. Again, this stands in contrast to the response of lymphocytes from patients with tuberculoid leprosy (Nogueira *et al.*, 1983). Thus, a state of relative IFN-γ deficiency may exist in the lesions of lepromatous leprosy. Moreover, monocytes from the lepromatous patients appear to secrete subnormal amounts of H_2O_2. Administration of very small doses of rIFN-γ into lepromatous lesions appears to correct this systemic defect, and possibly to activate intralesional mononuclear phagocytes as well (Nathan *et al.*, 1986). These observations remain to be confirmed in larger numbers of subjects infected by this and other facultative or obligate intracellular pathogens.

Meanwhile, work in the mouse has already confirmed that IFN-γ can activate macrophages *in vivo* in that species. The murine studies first recapitulated key points of the work *in vitro* described above with human cells and reagents. Thus, concanavalin A-stimulated mouse spleen cell supernatants augmented the H_2O_2-releasing capacity of resident mouse peritoneal macrophages, and this was abolished by monoclonal antibody against murine IFN-γ. Recombinant murine IFN-γ acted as a potent activating factor. These results with oxidative metabolism were recapitulated when we studied

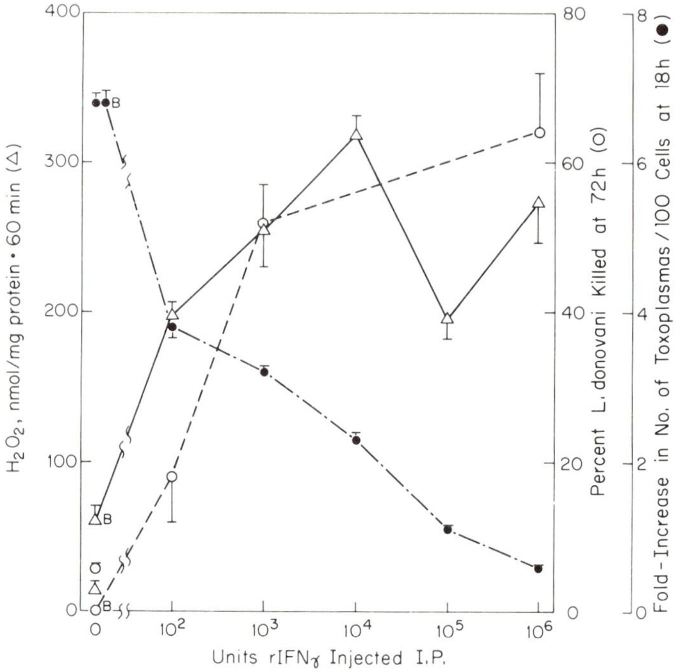

Fig. 1 Effect of injection of rIFN-γ-mu on the capacity of mouse peritoneal macrophages to release H_2O_2 (open triangles), inhibit the replication of *T. gondii* (closed circles), and kill *L. donovani* (open circles). Mice were injected i.p. with the indicated nominal number of antiviral units of rIFN-γ-mu (purified from transfected *E. coli* and provided by Genentech, Inc.) 18 hours before collection of peritoneal cells. The actual amount of rIFN-γ injected was less than the nominal amount, because of loss by adsorption to the syringe. Points marked "B" are results for mice injected with diluent alone. The other data for 0 units of rIFN-γ-mu are from uninjected mice. Reprinted from Murray, *et al.* (1985).

the ability of macrophages to kill *Toxoplasma gondii* and *Leishmania donovani* (Murray *et al.*, 1985). The concentrations of rIFN-γ required *in vitro* for half-maximal enhancement of these three features of macrophage function ranged from 0.03 to 0.14 antiviral unit per ml (sub-picomolar range).

A single intraperitoneal injection of rIFN-γ was administered to mice and peritoneal cells were collected 18 hours later. There was no effect of the injection on either the number or differential count of peritoneal cells. However, as illustrated in Fig. 1, the macrophages displayed dose-dependent increases in H_2O_2-releasing capacity and antiprotozoal activity, with half-maximal enhancement following the injection of 85–250 units (Murray *et al.*, 1985). The rIFN-γ was diluted in protein-free buffer and over 90% was lost by adherence to the tubes and syringes used for its administration. Thus, the amounts actually injected were probably far less than stated above. Peritoneal macrophages were also activated by administration of rIFN-γ by the intravenous or intramuscular routes (Murray *et al.*, 1985).

These results complement those showing reduction of counts of *Listeria monocytogenes* (Kiderlen *et al.*, 1984) or *Mycobacterium intracellulare* (Edwards *et al.*, 1985) or decreased mortality from *Toxoplasma gondii* in rIFN-γ-treated mice (McCabe *et al.*, 1984). Finally, Schreiber and his colleagues have demonstrated that administration of a monoclonal antibody to murine IFN-γ made mice succumb to otherwise self-limited listeriosis (Buchmeier and Schreiber, 1985).

From these studies, we conclude that IFN-γ is the predominant macrophage activating factor secreted by clonally unselected lymphocytes in at least two species; that this pertains both to splenic lymphocytes (in the mouse) and to peripheral blood lymphocytes (in man); that IFN-γ acts not only on macrophages derived *in vitro* from monocytes but also on tissue macrophages; that it is effective both *in vitro* and *in vivo*; and that its potency in both milieux is remarkable.

III REGULATION OF MACROPHAGE NEOPTERIN SECRETION BY IFN-γ

In bacteria, dihydroneopterin (2-amino-4-oxo-3,4-dihydro-6-trihydroxypropylpteridine) is an intermediate in the metabolism of GTP to folic acid (Brown and Williamson, 1982) (Fig. 2). In man, its precursor, neopterin triphosphate, is also the precursor of biopterin, a cofactor in the oxidation of phenylalanine, tyrosine, and tryptophan to dopamine and serotonin, and of glyceryl ethers to alcohols (Kaufman, 1967; Tietz *et al.*, 1964). Even though mammals cannot synthesize folate, neopterin is elevated in the plasma and urine of many human subjects with leprosy, tuberculosis, toxoplasmosis, malaria, renal allograft rejection, malignancies, viral infections, acquired immunodeficiency syndrome, and other inflammatory conditions (Margreiter *et al.*, 1983; Hausen and Wachter, 1982a; Wachter *et al.*, 1982; 1983). The biological significance of these elevated levels has not been readily appreciated and their clinical utility has not been fully realized in the absence of knowledge of the source of extracellular neopterin and the means of control of its secretion.

The elevation of neopterin in the urine of patients with malignancies led some investigators to assume that it arose from neoplastic cells. However, secretion of neopterin by transformed cells *in vitro* has apparently never been demonstrated. When renal allograft rejection was recognized as another setting for marked increases in urinary neopterin, it was stated

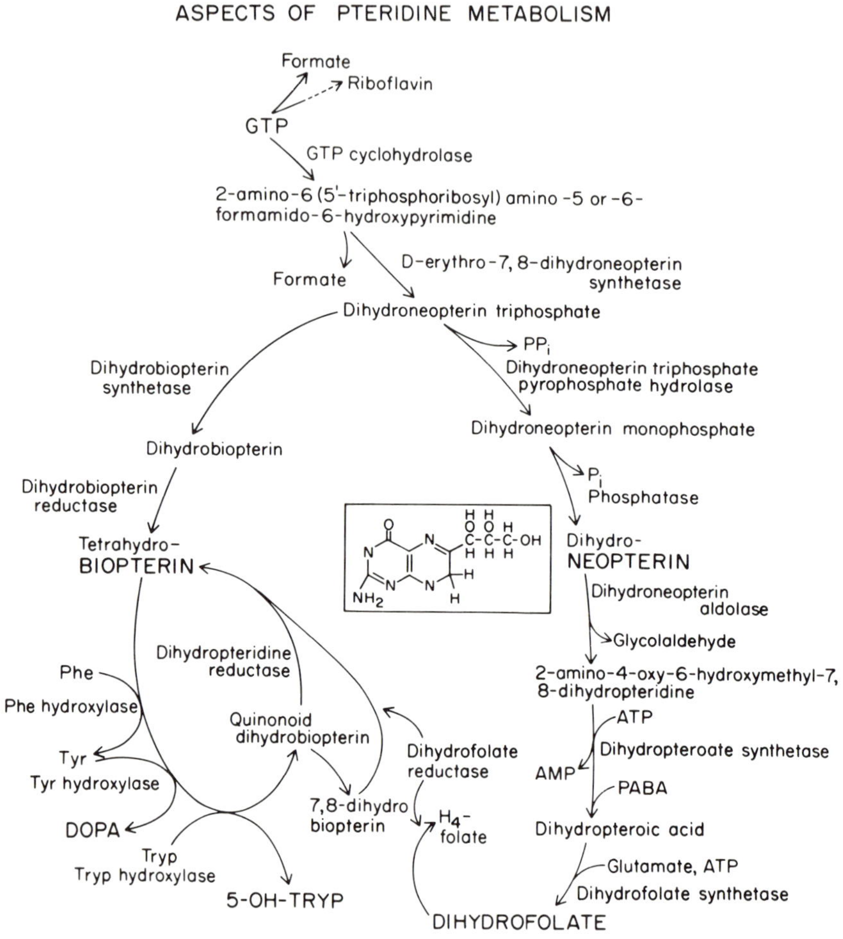

Fig. 2 Aspects of pteridine metabolism: a composite from different species, ranging from *E. coli* to man. Each species does not synthesize all the products indicated. The number of intermediate steps may also vary among species. Metal-ion cofactors are not shown.

to derive from T lymphocytes. This view was supported by the demonstration that neopterin accumulates in medium conditioned by mononuclear leukocytes reacting to allogeneic leukocytes or mitogenic lectins (Huber *et al.*, 1983). However, cloned T cells failed to release neopterin. It soon became apparent that antigen- or mitogen-stimulated T cells released a factor that induced neopterin secretion in mononuclear phagocytes. This T-cell-derived factor was neutralized by monoclonal antibody to IFN-γ and could be replaced by rIFN-γ (Huber *et al.*, 1984). T cells themselves, as well as B cells and large granular lymphocytes, secreted no detectable neopterin under the same conditions (Huber *et al.*, 1984).

While the work reported was in progress, a similar study was carried out in which I prepared media conditioned by human monocyte-derived macrophages in response to various cytokines and submitted them for neopterin assay to D. Fuchs, A. Hausen, G. Reibnegger and H. Wachter of the Department of Medical Chemistry and Biochemistry, University of Innsbruck, Innsbruck, Austria. The results confirm and extend those of Huber *et al.* and are summarized below.

Monocytes from venous blood of normal donors were cultured on glass coverslips as described (Nathan *et al.*, 1983a; Nakagawara *et al.*, 1981). On the 4th–6th day of culture, at which time less than 0.4% of the cells stained with fluoresceinated anti-Leu 4 monoclonal antibody, the indicated cytokines (characterized in Nathan *et al.*, 1984) were added in fresh medium (RPMI-1640 with antibiotics and 25% fresh-frozen human serum from donors of AB blood type) as reported. Three to four days later, the media were collected and stored at $-20°C$ until assay by HPLC, utilizing fluorescent detection of compounds eluting with authentic fully oxidized neopterin (Hausen *et al.*, 1982b). The cell-bearing coverslips were then washed and one set of triplicates used to measure adherent cell protein by the method of Lowry *et al.* (1951), while a second set of triplicates was used to measure H_2O_2 secretion in response to 100 ng/ml phorbol myristate acetate by the horseradish-peroxidase-mediated oxidation of fluorescent scopoletin (Nakagawara *et al.*, 1981). Ficoll-Hypaque purified mononuclear leukocytes nonadherent to plastic after 2–3 hours in the presence of 25% human serum were obtained from the same blood specimens that provided the monocytes and were incubated for the next 2–4 days in cytokines as indicated. Media were then assayed for neopterin as above. Fibroblasts from American Type Culture Collection, Rockville, MD, and carcinoma cell lines from Dr J. Fogh, Sloan-Kettering Institute, Rye, NY, were cultured in RPMI-1640 with 10% fetal bovine serum, penicillin, and streptomycin. Phenol-extracted *E. coli* lipopolysaccharide endotoxin (LPS) was a kind gift of Dr R. B. Johnston, Jr, National Jewish Hospital, Denver, CO. D-(+)-neopterin was purchased from Fluka Chemical Corp., Hauppague, NY.

As shown in Table V, rIFN-γ was the only one of seven cytokines tested that reliably induced neopterin secretion (96% of 57 cultures were positive, compared to 0–20% of cultures containing other cytokines). Neopterin levels in rIFN-γ-treated cultures averaged 39-fold higher than the medium control. In contrast to H_2O_2, neopterin was secreted without the addition of a secretagogue such as phorbol myristate acetate (PMA); nor did PMA augment its release (not shown). The only other agent tested that induced neopterin secretion was LPS. However, the effect of LPS was variable (Table V). The

TABLE V Secretion of Neopterin and H_2O_2 by Human Macrophages Incubated in Various Cytokines

Cytokine	Concentration (Units/ml)[b]	Neopterin (pmol/mg protein per 3–4 days)[c]	% Positive tests[a]	H_2O_2 (nmol/mg protein per 60 min)
none		19 ± 11 (13)[d]	19	49 ± 10[e]
rIFN-γ	10–1000	748 ± 148 (11)	96	341 ± 47
nIFN-α	1000–10,000	0 ± 0 (5)	0	40 ± 22
rIFN-αA	1000–10,000	0 ± 0 (4)	0	66 ± 33
rIFN-αD	1000–10,000	40 ± 53 (3)	13	20 ± 11
rIFN-β	1000–10,000	86 ± 81 (5)	18	65 ± 23
CSF-1	500	0 ± 0 (5)	0	21 ± 11
GM-CSF	500	0 ± 0 (6)	0	73 ± 33
LPS	10–100	173 ± 45 (3)	59	67 ± 19

[a] Percentage of all cultures tested in which neopterin was detectable.

[b] As defined in Nathan *et al.*, (1984) except for LPS, which is given in ng/ml.

[c] Limit of detection, 5 pmol/ml, corresponding to a mean of 100 pmol/mg protein (0.5 ml cultures with an average of 25 μg cell protein). Samples with undetectable neopterin were assigned a value of 0 for computation of means.

[d] Mean ± standard error for all cultures tested in the number of independent experiments in parentheses, each with a different donor.

[e] Following addition of PMA to the same cells whose culture medium was assayed for neopterin.

rIFN-γ used in these studies was negative for LPS by the limulus amoebocyte lysate test. Reagent neopterin, added to macrophages at the concentrations attained with rIFN-γ (1–100 nM), had no effect on H_2O_2 release, nor did it synergize with rIFN-γ in elevating H_2O_2-releasing capacity (not shown).

The concentrations of rIFN-γ required to activate macrophage oxidative metabolism and to induce neopterin secretion were closely comparable, when tested with the same cells (Fig. 3). In the experiments shown, 50% of maximal stimulation of neopterin secretion required $\sim 10^{-10}$ M rIFN-γ. Neopterin was detectable in the medium of macrophages within one day after addition of rIFN-γ, but reached higher levels by 3 days (not shown), as is the case for augmentation of H_2O_2 releasing capacity (Nathan *et al.*, 1983a). Freshly explanted monocytes also secreted neopterin if they were exposed to rIFN-γ (not shown). However, the same cells secreted abundant hydrogen peroxide without known exposure to IFN-γ *in vitro* (Nakagawara *et al.*, 1981). Thus, in the freshly cultured monocyte, secretion of neopterin appeared to correlate more closely with known prior exposure to IFN-γ than did capacity to secrete H_2O_2.

Induction of neopterin secretion was not a feature of IFN-γ action on other cell types, including lymphocytes and granulocytes from the same blood

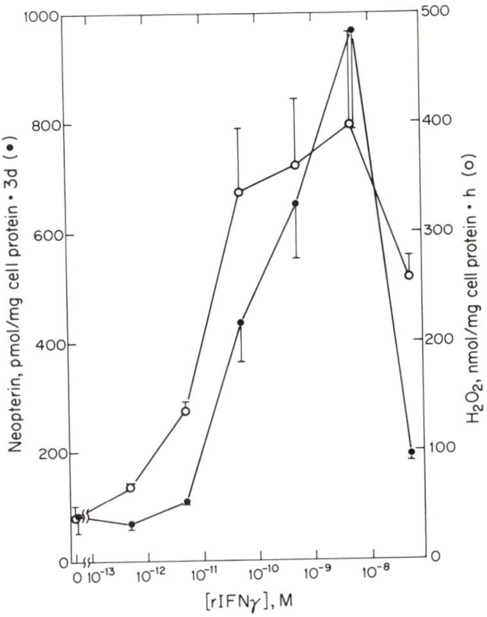

Fig. 3 Macrophages were cultured with pure recombinant IFN-γ (Genentech, Inc., South San Francisco, CA) for 3 days and the media assayed for neopterin. The cells were then stimulated to secrete H_2O_2 by addition of PMA, as described in Table I. Means $\pm$ standard errors from two experiments.

samples that provided the macrophages (Table VI). None of the normal mesenchymal or malignant epithelial human cell lines tested secreted detectable neopterin, with or without exposure to IFNs (Table VI).

From these results it appears that human monocyte-derived macrophages, but not granulocytes, blood lymphocytes, cultured fibroblasts, ovarian carcinoma cells, or breast carcinoma cells, secrete copious oxidized neopterin *in vitro* after exposure to rIFN-γ. Little or no oxidized neopterin was secreted by macrophages in the absence of IFN-γ, or in the presence of a mixture of native IFN-α's, or rIFN-α types A or D, rIFN-β, CSF-1, or GM-CSF. In contrast, Huber *et al.* (1984) did observe neopterin secretion by human monocytes in response to high concentrations of rIFN-α. The reasons for this difference are not known, but may relate to the IFN preparation used or the state of differentiation of the cells. In the present studies, LPS was variably effective at inducing neopterin secretion from macrophages *in vitro*, and may have been a contaminant of the media in which neopterin secretion was occasionally detected in the absence of rIFN-γ.

In its regulation by rIFN-γ, and in the dose requirements and time course of response to rIFN-γ, secretion of oxidized neopterin correlated with

TABLE VI Lack of Neopterin Secretion by Human Cells Other Than Macrophages[a]

Cells	Cytokine[b]	Neopterin (pmol/mg protein/2–4 days)[c]
Nonadherent blood mononuclear cells (mostly lymphocytes)	none	0 ± 0 (18)[d]
	rIFN-γ	6 ± 5 (18)[e]
Polymorphonuclear leukocytes	none	0 ± 0 (5)
	rIFN-γ	0 ± 0 (5)
Fibroblasts (normal diploid)	none	0 ± 0 (6)
	rIFN-γ	0 ± 0 (6)
	rIFN-αA	0 ± 0 (6)
	rIFN-β	0 ± 0 (6)
SK-OV3 (ovarian carcinoma)	none	0 ± 0 (6)
	rIFN-γ	0 ± 0 (6)
	rIFN-αA	0 ± 0 (6)
	rIFN-β	0 ± 0 (6)
CAMA (breast carcinoma)	none	0 ± 0 (6)
	rIFN-γ	0 ± 0 (6)
	rIFN-αA	0 ± 0 (6)
	rIFN-β	0 ± 0 (6)

[a] Positive controls were provided by experiments in Table V employing the same cytokine preparations and adherent cells from the same blood samples used here.

[b] 10–1000 U/ml of rIFN-γ, 500 U/ml of rIFN-αA, or 2500 U/ml of rIFN-β.

[c] Limit of detection 5 pmol/ml, corresponding to a mean of 26 pmol/mg protein for fibroblasts and tumour cells (1 ml cultures with an average of 189 μg cell protein). Nonadherent mononuclear cells and polymorphonuclear leukocytes were cultured at 2×10^6 cells/well in 0.5 ml.

[d] Mean ± standard error for the number of cultures in parentheses.

[e] Assuming 55 μg protein/10^6 cells.

capacity of mononuclear phagocytes to secrete H_2O_2. However, secretion of large amounts of H_2O_2 by macrophages is a two-step process: activation must be followed by a stimulus for secretion, such as interaction with microorganisms, immune complexes, or soluble secretagogues (Nathan and Root, 1977). In contrast, exposure to IFN-γ was the only apparent requirement for induction of oxidized neopterin secretion from macrophages. However, small amounts of H_2O_2 are secreted by activated macrophages *in vitro* even without a known stimulus of the respiratory burst (Nathan and Klebanoff, 1982). Thus, it is possible that reactive oxygen intermediates are responsible for converting dihydroneopterin to the oxidized, fluorescent form that is detected by the assay used. It is also highly likely that the total amount of neopterin produced (reduced plus oxidized) is elevated in the IFN-γ-treated human mononuclear phagocyte. It remains to be demonstrated precisely how much of the increase in detectable neopterin induced by rIFN-γ is due to augmented synthesis, increased oxidation, or decreased catabolism, whether the responsible reactions are enzymatic, and, if so, whether the enzymes are induced, activated, or inhibited by IFN-γ treatment.

It also remains to be established how much of the elevation in plasma and urinary neopterin in inflammatory states can be attributed to macrophages and how much to other cell types that have not yet been tested. Finally, not all the clinical states associated with elevated neopterin are likely settings for IFN-γ action. Notably, the acquired immunodeficiency syndrome, in which IFN-γ secretion is abnormally low, is associated with some of the highest neopterin levels, and in this case other regulatory factors are likely to be at work. Nonetheless, the possibility deserves further study that urinary neopterin may be a useful monitor of IFN-γ effect *in vivo* in selected situations.

IV IFN-γ AND THE ANTIMICROBIAL STATE: A HYPOTHESIS

Is neopterin synthesized in man as a waste product? Or is there some benefit to the host in having its macrophages (and possibly other cells) convert considerable GTP into oxidized neopterin whenever T cells or NK cells respond to foreign antigens by secreting IFN-γ? In accord with the premise that IFN-γ's chief physiological role may be the induction of antibacterial, antiprotozoal and antifungal states in parasitized cells, an interesting possibility is that oxidized neopterin may function to inhibit folate synthesis by intracellular pathogenic microorganisms. Figure 2 illustrates the pathways under discussion.

Some of the earliest studies of folate synthesis by bacterial lysates demonstrated a requirement for reducing conditions, such as NADH, 2-mercaptoethanol, and a nitrogen atmosphere (Brown, 1959). The basis for this requirement was elucidated with the subsequent demonstration that at least two enzymes in the folate synthetic path require the pteridine substrate to be in the dihydro form. Thus, dihydroneopterin aldolase will not use oxidized neopterin to produce the 2-amino-4-hydroxy-6-hydroxymethyl-7,8-dihydropteridine required by dihydropteroic acid synthetase (Mathis and Brown, 1970). The latter enzyme will not use oxidized 2-amino-4-hydroxy-6-hydroxymethylpteridine in the condensation with *p*-aminobenzoic acid (PABA) (Shiota and Disraely, 1961). Although the oxidized forms of the substrates have apparently not been tested directly as inhibitors of the reactions with the dihydro forms, it is possible that they would exert such an effect on one or both of these enzymes, in addition to competition by dilution of the pool of reduced substrates. There is a related example: oxidation of the pteridine nucleus of pteroylpolyglutamates increases their capacity to inhibit thymidylate synthetase (Kisliuk *et al.*, 1974).

Sulfonamides were the first antimetabolite antimicrobials, and the first drugs to cure systemic bacterial infections in man. Through their structural resemblance to PABA, they inhibit its incorporation into dihydropteroic acid. This may occur both by diluting the pool of PABA that can be utilized by the enzyme, and also by serving as a substrate that forms an adduct with 2-amino-4-hydroxy-6-hydroxymethyl-7,8-dihydropteridine which cannot be further metabolized by the next enzyme in the pathway, dihydrofolate synthetase (Brown and Williamson, 1982). If oxidized neopterin decreases the utilization of dihydropteridine substrates by either dihydroneopterin aldolase or dihydropteroate synthetase—whether by competition or by inhibition—it might exert a microbistatic action similar to that of sulfonamides, inhibiting many (but not all) of those microorganisms that must synthesize their own folic acid and cannot utilize the exogenous compound. At the same time, oxidized neopterin would be expected to pose no threat to host cells, which cannot synthesize folate and instead depend on the exogenous vitamin.

By analogy with sulfonamides, the spectrum of microbistatic action of oxidized neopterin might include a number of the facultative intracellular pathogens that tend to persist within resident tissue macrophages but are eliminated by immunologically activated macrophages, such as species of *Corynebacteria, Brucella, Pasteurella, Nocardia*, and *Chlamydia*. In the case of sulfonamide-resistant facultative intracellular pathogens of macrophages, such as *Mycobacteria*, *Rickettsia*, and *Candida*, a possible role of oxidized neopterin cannot be discounted without knowing the basis of sulfonamide resistance. In addition to capacity to utilize exogenous folate, sulfonamide resistance can reflect enhanced capacity to synthesize PABA, decreased sulfonamide uptake, or increased sulfonamide catabolism. In the latter three cases, oxidized neopterin might still exert an antimicrobial action. In this regard, it is of particular interest that *Mycobacteria* and *Plasmodia*, which are resistant to sulfonamides, are generally sensitive to sulfones, such as diaminodiphenylsulfone (dapsone), itself an inhibitor of dihyropteroate synthetase (McCoullugh and Maren, 1974). Thus, sulfonamide resistance does not always exclude a role for inhibition of folate synthesis as a mechanism of microbistasis.

According to this hypothesis, reactive oxygen intermediates produced by IFN-γ-activated macrophages may play at least two antimicrobial roles. The respiratory burst may kill a proportion of microorganisms during their ingestion. Low-level production of oxidants thereafter may serve to maintain neopterin in the oxidized state, contributing to inhibition of growth of surviving organisms.

Lymphokine (probably IFN-γ) enhances the activity of respiratory-burst-independent antimicrobial mechanisms in macrophages (Pfefferkorn, 1984; Murray *et al.*, 1983b). It is important to keep in mind that even if neopterin production proves to be one such mechanism, others are likely to exist as well (Elsbach and Weiss, 1983).

There is no reason why this postulated role of oxidized neopterin should be limited to macrophages, if other IFN-γ-responsive cells can both produce neopterin and oxidize it. Hepatocytes harbouring plasmodia (cited in Vilček *et al.*, 1985) and endothelial cells infected by rickettsia (Wisseman and Waddell, 1983) can eliminate the parasites in response to IFN-γ. The mechanisms of antimicrobial activity in these and other physiologically important settings involving non-phagocytic cells are completely unknown.

One pteridine-dependent, IFN-γ-induced antiprotozoal mechanism has already been elucidated. This is the enhancement of indoleamine dioxygenase activity in human fibroblasts by IFN-γ, leading to degradation of tryptophan in the culture medium and the consequent inhibition of replication of intracellular *Toxoplasma gondii* (Pfefferkorn, 1984). Indoleamine dioxygenase requires biopterin as a cofactor. In some tissues, biopterin is rate-limiting in the enzymatic reactions in which it is involved (Viveros *et al.*, 1981). However, it is not known whether biopterin is rate-limiting for indoleamine dioxygenase in human fibroblasts, nor whether they produce biopterin in response to IFN-γ. Thus, the precise level at which IFN-γ enhances indoleamine dioxygenase activity in fibroblasts remains to be determined. Furthermore, IFN-γ-activated macrophages readily kill *T. gondii.* There is no evidence that macrophages produce biopterin, and the indoleamine dioxygenase activity of macrophages is not enhanced by IFN-γ (E. Pfefferkorn, personal communication). Finally, tryptophan supplied at the level found in plasma completely reverses the toxoplasmastatic effect of tryptophan depletion in cell culture (Pfefferkorn 1984). Thus, induction of indoleamine dioxygenase activity is neither a general feature of IFN-γ-induced antitoxoplasma activity nor likely to be an effective antitoxoplasma mechanism in tissues whose extracellular fluid tryptophan readily equilibrates with tryptophan in plasma.

In conclusion, it seems likely that IFN-γ induces a variety of antibacterial, antiprotozoal and antifungal actions in a diversity of parasitized host cells. Enhanced secretion of reactive oxygen intermediates by macrophages is one such mechanism. Enhanced production of oxidized neopterin may be another, but this remains to be tested. If neopterin indeed proves to be an IFN-γ-induced antibiotic with a mechanism of action analogous to that of sulfas, it will not be the only time that one of man's most ingenious drugs is found to have been invented first by evolution.

ACKNOWLEDGEMENTS

I thank T. Prendergast for expert assistance and J. Leibowitch for introducing me to the subject of pteridines. Genentech and Hoffman-La Roche supplied interferons, and E. R. Stanley, E. Platzer, and K. Welte provided CSFs. Neopterin assays were performed by D. Fuchs, A. Hausen, G. Reibnegger and H. Wachter.

Note added in proof: Preliminary experiments by David Campanelli in the author's laboratory have not revealed an antibiotic effect of oxidized neopterin.

REFERENCES

Brown, G. M. (1959). *Fed. Proc.* **18**, 19 (abstract).
Brown, G. M. and Williamson, J. M. (1982). *Adv. Enzymol.* **53**, 345.
Buchmeier, N. A. and Schreiber, R. D. (1985). *Proc. Natl. Acad. Sci. USA* **82**, 7404.
Byrne, G. I. and Krueger, D. A. (1983). *Infect. Immunol.* **42**, 1152.
Edwards, C. K. III, Hedegaard, H. B., Zlotnik, A., Gangadharam, T. R., Johnston, R. B. Jr. and Pabst, M. J. (1985). *J. Immunol.* **136**, 1820.
Elsbach, P. and Weiss, J. (1983). *Rev. Infect. Dis.* **5**, 843.
Fowles, R. E., Fajardo, I. M., Leibowitch, J. L., and David, J. R. (1973). *J. Exp. Med.* **138**, 952.
de la Harpe, J. and Nathan, C. F. (1985). *J. Immunol. Meth.* **78**, 323.
Hausen, A. and Wachter, H. (1982a). *J. Clin. Chem. Clin. Biochem.* **20**, 593.
Hausen, A., Fuchs, D., Konig, K. and Wachter, H. (1982b). *J. Chromatogr.* **227**, 61.
Horwitz, M. A. (1985). Lecture, Trudeau Institute Workshop on Cell-Mediated Immunity, July 1985.
Horwitz, M. A., Levis, W. R. and Cohn, Z. A. (1984). *J. Exp. Med.* **159**, 666.
Huber, C., Fuchs, D., Hausen, A., Margreiter, R., Reibnegger, G., Spielberger, M. and Wachter, H. (1983). *J. Immunol.* **130**, 1047.
Huber, C., Batchelor, J. R., Fuchs, D., Hausen, A., Lang, A., Niederwieser, D., Reibnegger, G., Swetly, P., Troppmair, J. and Wachter, H. (1984). *J. Exp. Med.* **160**, 310.
Kaufman, S. (1967). *Ann. Rev. Biochem.* **36**, 171.
Kiderlen, A. F., Kaufmann, S. H. E. and Lohmann-Matthes M.-L. (1984). *Eur. J. Immunol.* **14**, 964.
Kisliuk, R. L., Gaumont, Y. and Baugh, C. M. (1974). *J. Biol. Chem.* **249**, 4100.
Lowry, O. H., Rosebrough, N. J., Farr, A. L. and Randall, R. J. (1951). *J. Biol. Chem.* **193**, 265.
McCabe, R. E., Luft, B. J. and Remington, J. S. (1984). *J. Infect. Dis.* **150**, 961.
McCoullugh, J. L. and Maren, T. H. (1974). *Molec. Pharmacol.* **10**, 140.
Mackaness, G. B. (1970). *In* "Infectious Agents and Host Reactions" (S. Mudd, ed.) pp 61–75. W. B. Saunders Co., Philadelphia.
Margreiter, R., Fuchs, D., Hausen, A., Huber, C., Reibnegger, G., Spielberger, M. and Wachter, H. (1983). *Transplantation* **36**, 650.
Mathis, J. B. and Brown, G. M. (1970). *J. Biol. Chem.* **245** 3015.
Murray, H. W., Rubin, B. Y. and Rothermel, C. D. (1983a). *J. Clin. Invest.* **72**, 1506.

Murray, H. W., Byrne, G. I., Rothermel, C. D. and Cartelli, D. M. (1983b). *J. Exp. Med.* **158**, 234.
Murray, H. W., Spitalny, G. and Nathan, C. F. (1985). *J. Immunol.* **134**, 1619.
Nakagawara, A., Nathan, C. F. and Cohn, Z. A. (1981). *J. Clin. Invest.* **68**, 1243.
Nathan, C. F. and Tsunakawi, S. (1986). *In* "Biochemistry of Macrophages" (D. Evered, J. Nugent, and M. O'Connor, eds.). Pitman, London.
Nathan, C. F., Karnovsky, M. L. and David, J. R. (1971). *J. Exp. Med.* **133**, 1356.
Nathan, C. F., Remold, H. G. and David, J. R. (1973). *J. Exp. Med.* **137**, 275.
Nathan, C. F. and Root, R. K. (1977). *J. Exp. Med.* **146**, 1648.
Nathan, C. F. and Klebanoff, S. J. (1982). *J. Exp. Med.* **155**, 1291.
Nathan, C. F., Murray, H. W., Wiebe, M. E. and Rubin, B. Y. (1983a). *J. Exp. Med.* **158**, 670.
Nathan, C. F. (1983b). *Trans. R. Soc. Trop. Med. Hyg.* **77**, 620.
Nathan, C. F., Prendergast, T. J., Wiebe, M. E., Stanley, E. R., Platzer, E., Remold, H. G., Welte, K., Rubin, B. Y. and Murray, H. W. (1984). *J. Exp. Med.* **160**, 600.
Nathan, C. F., Horowitz, C. R., de la Harpe, J., Vadhan-Raj, S., Sherwin, S. A., Oettgen, H. E. and Krown, S. E. (1985). *Proc. Natl. Acad. Sci. USA*. (in press).
Nathan, C. F., Kaplan, G., Levis, W., Nusrat, A., Witmer, M., Sherwin, S., Job, C. K., Horowitz, C. R., Steinman, R. and Cohn, Z. (1986) *N. Engl. J. Med.* in press.
Nogueira, N., Kaplan, G., Levy, E., Sarno, E. N., Kushner, P., Granelli-Piperno, A. Viera, L., Colomer-Gould, V., Levis, W., Steinman, R., Yip, Y. K., and Cohn, Z. (1983). *J. Exp. Med.* **158**, 2165.
Ockenhouse, C. F., Schulman, S. and Shear, H. L. (1984). *J. Immunol.* **133**, 1601.
Peck, R. (1985). *J. Immunolog. Meth.* **82**, 131.
Pfefferkorn, E. R. (1984). *Proc. Natl Acad. Sci. USA* **81**, 908.
Plata, F., Wietzerbin, J., Pons, F. G., Falcoff, E. and Eisen, H. (1984). *Eur. J. Immunol.* **14**, 930.
Rothermel, C. D., Rubin, B. Y., and Murray, H. W. (1983). *J. Immunol.* **131**, 2542.
Schreiber, R. D., Hicks, L. J., Celada, A., Buchmeier, N. A. and Gray, P. W. (1985). *J. Immunol.* **134**: 1609.
Shiota, T. and Disraely, M. N. (1961). *Biochim. Biophys. Acta* **52**, 467.
Stone-Wolff, D. S., Yip, Y. K., Chroboczek-Kelker, H., Henriksen-DeStefano, J. Le, D., Rubin, B. Y., Rinderknecht, E., Aggarwal, B. B., and Vilček, J. (1984). *J. Exp. Med.* **159**, 828.
Tietz, A., Lindberg, M. and Kennedy, E. P. (1964). *J. Biol. Chem.* **239**: 4081.
Turco, J. and Winkler, H. H. (1983). *J. Exp. Med.* **158**, 2159.
Vilček, J., Gray, P. W., Rinderknecht, E. and Sevastopoulos, C. G., (1985). *Lymphokines* **11**, 1.
Viveros, O. H., Lee, C.-L., Abou-Donia, M. M., Nixon, J. C. and Nichol, C. A. (1981). *Science* **213**, 349.
Wachter, H., Curtius, H. C., and Pfleiderer, W. (eds.) (1982). "Biochemical and Clinical Aspects of Pteridines," Vol. 1, W. de Gruyter, Berlin.
Wachter, H., Fuchs, D., Hausen, A., Huber, C., Knosp, O., Reibnegger, G. and Spira, T. J. (1983). *Hoppe-Seyler's Z. Physiol. Chem.* **364**, 1345.
Wing, E. J., Ampel, N. M., Waheed, A. and Shadduck, R. K. (1985). *J. Immunol.* **135**, 2052.
Wirth, J. J., Kierszenbaum, F., Sonnenfeld, G. and Zlotnik, A. (1985). *Infect. Immunol.* **49**, 61.
Wisseman, C. L., Jr. and Waddell, A. (1983). *J. Exp. Med.* **157**, 1780.
Wu-Hsieh, B., Zlotnik, A., and Howard, D. H. (1984). *Infect. Immunol.* **43**, 380.

Interferon and the Tumour Cell Phenotype

DANIÈLE BROUTY-BOYÉ

Laboratory of Viral Oncology, Institut de Recherches Scientifiques sur le Cancer, BP 8, 94802 Villejuif, France

---

I INTRODUCTION

It has been thought for many years that the heritable cellular changes responsible for the tumorous state are irreversibly fixed. Various experimental facts, however, suggest that the malignant process is reversible. There are several reports defining the conditions of cell culture that affect the phenotypic properties of transformed and tumorigenic cells so that they behave as normal cells (reviewed in Topp *et al.*, 1980). In agreement with these studies were our observations that during serial passages at low cell density, the phenotype of murine x-ray-transformed 10T1/2 cells progressively changed and eventually displayed characteristics of untransformed cells (Brouty-Boyé *et al.*, 1979). A critical question at that time was whether the conditions of culture that we and others employed allowed for the selective proliferation of untransformed cells. By cloning the reverted

INTERFERON 7
ISBN 0 12 302256 8

cells and repassaging them at high cell density, we found that they rapidly regained their transformed and tumorigenic properties (Brouty-Boyé *et al.*, 1982a). This result suggested that reversion did not arise by selection of pre-existing variants but implied that a modulation of the transformed phenotype had been achieved by the conditions of culture to which these cells were exposed. Another example illustrating that tumour cells can be manipulated to attain a normal phenotype is that of a highly malignant transplantable teratocarcinoma of the mouse which can convert to normal when placed in the appropriate microenvironment *in vivo* (Mintz and Illmensee, 1975).

From these intriguing phenomena and the recently advanced knowledge of tumour cell origins, there is reason to believe that physiological or non-physiological substances exist that can redirect tumour cells toward a normal stage. Our first experimental approach using IFN and x-ray-transformed cells indicated that this naturally occuring substance might in fact induce phenotypic reversion. These findings generated further investigations in different cell systems in an attempt to determine whether normalization of tumour cells might well be one of the effective actions of IFNs on tumour growth *in vivo*.

II INTERFERON-INDUCED REVERSION IN X-RAY-TRANSFORMED 10T1/2 CELLS

When we started our work in 1979, there were several fragmentary reports suggesting that IFN might induce changes in the cell phenotype. In the early 1960s it was noted that a change in the morphology of human amniotic cells occurred when treated with IFN (Gresser, 1961). Later it was shown that IFN treatment *in vitro* reduced the proliferation and the ability of different tumour cells to form colonies in soft agar or tumours in animals (reviewed in Brouty-Boyé, 1980). Even *in vivo*, it was noted in earlier studies that the spleens of mice infected with Friend leukemia virus and treated with IFN contained more extensive areas of erythroid maturation than the spleens of untreated leukemic mice (Gresser *et al.*, 1967). The idea that IFN could alter the cell phenotype received further support from the description of IFN's effects on various cell functions of both normal and malignant cells (reviewed in Taylor-Papadimitriou, 1982).

In different cell systems most of these effects were detected within a few days of IFN treatment. It is curious that many of the investigations of the non-antiviral activities of IFN *in vitro* concentrated on the effects of short-term treatment even though long-term IFN therapy proved to be more efficient in experimental *in vivo* models (Gresser, 1977). The studies *in vitro* dealing with the long-term subcultivation of cells in the continuous presence of IFN were mostly directed at the selection of resistant cells. It was evident that information was lacking with respect to the long-term effect of IFN on the transformed cell phenotype. There was, however, one reported attempt to investigate this question. Chany and Vignal in 1970 showed that when murine embryo-fibroblasts transformed by Moloney sarcoma virus were serially cultivated in the presence of IFN for extended periods, the cells regained some of the characteristics of untransformed cells. The sequence of events preceding these changes, however, was not investigated. The cells were characterized only after having been passaged for more than 200 times in the presence of IFN.

Our studies using 10T1/2 cells transformed by x-irradiation focused on characterizing the early specific cellular changes, which eventually lead to the reversal of the transformed and tumorigenic phenotype. In these studies, mouse C243 cell IFN-α/β was used either partially purified (specific activity of 1 to 2.9 $\times$ 10^7 units/mg of proteins (Tovey *et al.*, 1974)) or highly purified (specific activity of 5 $\times$ 10^8 to 1 $\times$ 10^9 units/mg of proteins (De Maeyer-Guignard *et al.*, 1978; Aguet, 1980)) at a dose of 640 units. The passage of transformed cells was performed once every week at seeding concentrations known to be high enough to retain the transformed and tumorigenic phenotype (10^4 cells/cm^2).

We observed modifications leading to the restoration of more normal properties when two clones of x-ray-transformed cells were continuously exposed to IFN (Table I) (Brouty-Boyé and Gresser, 1981; Brouty-Boyé *et al.*, 1982b). An important finding was the progressive appearance of the cellular changes.

There was an immediate inhibitory effect on cellular proliferation within 24 hours of IFN treatment, which was mediated by a reduced growth rate and saturation density at values nearly that of parental untransformed 10T1/2 cells. Surprisingly, growth inhibitory effects progressively decreased even in the presence of 100-fold higher doses of IFN. However, during this time, no change was detected in the sensitivity of the cells to the antiviral activity of IFN. The reduced sensitivity to the antiproliferative but not to the antiviral activity that developed during long-term treatment clearly indicated a difference in IFN's effects on these two processes. It should be mentioned that this refractory state was reversible after several cell passages in the absence of IFN (Brouty-Boyé, 1982).

In contrast to the immediate inhibition of cell proliferation, the changes in cellular morphology and tumorigenicity did not occur during the first

TABLE I Phenotypic Characteristics of C3H/10T1/2 Cell Lines

Untransformed cells	X-ray-transformed cells	
No treatment	No treatment	Long-term IFN treatment
Flat epithelioid morphology	Fibroblastic-like morphology	Flat epithelioid or elongated morphology
Adhesiveness	Disruption of microfilament bundles	Organized microfilament bundles
Density-dependent growth inhibition	Decreased adhesion plaques	Abundant adhesion plaques
Anchorage-dependent growth	Decreased adhesiveness	Increased adhesiveness
High sensitivity to IFN	Loss of density-dependent growth inhibition	Loss of cell piling
Lack of tumorigenicity	Acquisition of anchorage-independent growth	Low sensitivity to IFN
	Decreased sensitivity to IFN	Loss of tumorigenicity
	Tumorigenicity	

passage with IFN. They progressively appeared on further passage with IFN.*

Regarding the morphology, it was only after seven passages that IFN-treated clones assumed a flattened morphology, either epithelioid in one clone (Fig. 1C) or elongated and well-orientated (Fig. 1D) in the other, with no cellular overlapping, whereas both untreated cells displayed fibroblastic-like morphology with extensive cellular overlapping (Fig. 1B). Another aspect of the morphological changes was the increased adhesiveness of the treated transformed cells to the plastic substrate.

We found that changes reminiscent of normal cells, in the morphology and in the adhesiveness of IFN-treated x-ray-transformed cells, were associated with changes in those elements of the cytoskeleton that were nearly absent in transformed cells (Brouty-Boyé *et al.*, 1981); i.e. submembranous and cytoplasmic microfilaments and vinculin-containing plaques. There was extensive development of microtubules and intermediate filaments and elevated expression of fibronectin in both treated and untreated cells. Therefore, the entire submembranous and cytoplasmic network of microfilaments and their related junctional structures to the membrane appeared extensively developed under IFN treatment. It is likely that these effects are intimately related to the slowdown in cell proliferation, decrease in saturation density, increase in cell adhesiveness and overall changes in cell morphology.

Similar to the reversal of cell morphology, the reduction in the tumorigenicity of x-ray-transformed cells was progressive to a point of apparent extinction. The duration of this process was, however, much longer. It was only after 24 passages (a 6-month treatment) that the cells no longer induced tumours in mice. The loss of tumorigenicity was repeatedly obtained using close to 100 mice.

In view of the *progressive* and *sequential* nature of the reversion, the question arises "Why is such a high number of passages required for reversion to be fully expressed?" Does this imply that reverted cells arise from selection of pre-existing variants or does it indicate that a series of regulatory changes is required to revert the multistep process of transformation? The first possibility, selection, appears unlikely for at least two reasons. (1) Reversion was obtained in transformed cells cloned twice, which should exclude the existence of a mixed-cell population. (2) IFN-treated cells retained the potential to back-revert to their initial transformed phenotype

* Since these changes occurred during the period refractory to the antiproliferative effects of IFN, it is unlikely that it was inhibition of cell proliferation *per se* that led to the various changes in transformed properties. In support of this, it has been shown that substitution of the protein inhibitor cycloheximide, for IFN, in the serial passage of x-ray-transformed cells, induced a constant reduced proliferation, reversion of morphology, but no change in tumorigenicity (Brouty-Boyé and Gresser, 1981).

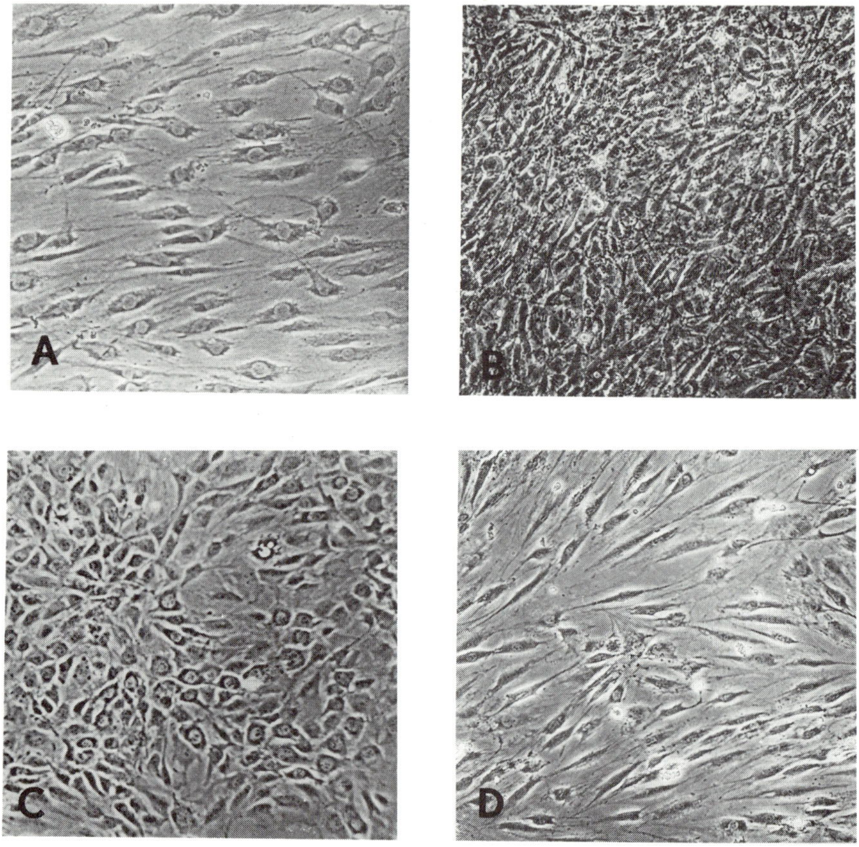

Fig. 1 Morphological reversion of x-ray-transformed C3H/10T1/2 cells under long-term treatment with IFN. (**A**) Untransformed 10T1/2 cells; (**B**) untreated x-ray-transformed cells; (**C**) transformed $5T_1$ and (**D**) $5T_3$ cells treated for more than 10 passages with IFN.

upon removal of IFN. Selection, however, cannot be ruled out, if only certain cells in the population of transformed cells have the potential to undergo reversion. If so, the prolonged duration of IFN treatment would give a selective advantage to the emergence of these cells. A selection of this type, however, does not exclude the second possibility of a *stepwise process*. The continuous presence of IFN may be looked upon as persistently activating those different events that are concerned with the suppression of transformed properties. Such a process may, in fact, evolve as one occurring in the generation of normal cells. In the course of their life cycle, normal cells pass through different stages in response to specific signals. Since tumour cells appear to retain the potential for behaving as normal cells, IFN might re-program the crucial events leading to the suppression of the transformed phenotype.

That IFN acts as a persistent signal fits well with the finding that *reversion is reversible*. If reversion is progressive, so is back-reversion. Thus, the return of the transformed phenotype is evident first at the level of cell growth, then of morphology, and much later for tumorigenicity.

III IS INTERFERON-INDUCED REVERSION A GENERAL PHENOMENON?

Since 10T1/2 cells were easily transformed by chemical carcinogens and oncogenic viruses, a comparison could be made between 10T1/2 cells transformed by different means and their response to IFN. Using experimental conditions similar to those employed in the treatment of x-ray-transformed cells, we investigated the long-term effects of IFN on 10T1/2 cells transformed by methylcholanthrene (MCA) and SV_{40}.*

The phenotypic characteristics of cloned MCA and SV_{40}-transformed 10T1/2 cells resembled those of x-ray-transformed cells based on criteria of cell proliferation, cell morphology, cell adhesiveness, cell structure, and ability to form colonies in soft agar. Their tumorigenic phenotype, however, differed. MCA-transformed cells grew faster and at a cell inoculum 100 times lower than x-ray-transformed cells, when implanted into nude or syngeneic C3H mice. Secondly, whereas MCA and x-ray-transformed cells gave rise to 100% tumours within one to three weeks after inoculation into nude mice, the tumour incidence of SV_{40}-transformed cells was only 20%.

Our results show that the same cell type transformed by different means displays different sensitivities to the numerous phenotypic changes induced by IFN (Brouty-Boyé *et al.*, 1984). With respect to the inhibition of cell proliferation, IFN initially reduced the rate of growth of both MCA and SV_{40}-transformed cells. Moreover, while MCA-transformed cell cultures reached low cell density with no cellular overlapping. SV_{40}-transformed cells became confluent at the same high density as untreated cultures and developed extensive cell piling. As observed for IFN-treated x-ray-transformed cells, growth inhibitory effects of IFN progressively decreased in MCA-transformed cells but persisted in SV_{40}-transformed cells.

In the presence of IFN, MCA-transformed cells appeared progressively flat and finally assumed an epithelioid morphology after several cell passages. Additionally, structural changes were evident in the appearance of a thick

* We chose this oncogenic DNA virus because early reports did not show any effects of IFN on the phenotypic characteristics of SV_{40}-transformed cells (Oxman *et al.*, 1967). At that time IFN effects other than antiviral were not well understood or well received.

layer of submembranous microfilaments. In contrast, the morphology of SV_{40}-transformed cells cultivated in the presence of even 100-fold higher doses of IFN did not significantly change.* It appears, therefore, that long-term treatment induces the reversal of the transformed properties of both x-ray and MCA-transformed cells on the basis of cell proliferation and cell morphology, without significantly modifying those of SV_{40}-transformed cells.

As to the tumorigenic properties, we found that the modifications brought about by IFN were much more pronounced in x-ray transformed cells than in MCA and SV_{40}-transformed cells.

In contrast to IFN-treated x-ray-transformed cells, suppression of the tumorigenic phenotype was not obtained in MCA-transformed cells. Although the rate of tumour growth and tumour appearance was delayed, the incidence of tumours in syngeneic C3H mice inoculated with IFN-treated MCA-transformed cells was not decreased. When injected into nude mice only a decrease in the rate of tumour growth was observed. The delay in tumour appearance observed in C3H, but not athymic, nude mice indicated that MCA-treated cells were more susceptible to T-cell-mediated host immune response than untreated cells. Similar results have been shown with murine MCA sarcoma cells treated *in vitro* with IFN (Wyvel and Pitha, 1982). In this latter study, the alterations in the tumour phenotype were induced by short-term IFN treatment and correlated with a decrease in the expression of the tumour-specific-transplantation antigen (TSTA) and an increase in H2-antigens that play a role in host recognition of the TSTA of MCA-induced sarcoma. If modifications in the tumorigenic phenotype are mainly mediated by the relatively rapid increase in cellular antigenicity, why, then, is long-term IFN treatment required to suppress the tumorigenic potential of x-ray-transformed cells? Moreover, since these cells were tested in nude mice, an increase in cellular antigenicity would play only a small part in their inability to grow in nude mice. These observations suggest that additional changes in tumour cell phenotype other than reduced proliferation, altered morphology and increased antigenicity contribute to the process of reversion.

One puzzling result is that in contrast to x-ray- and MCA-transformed cells, the tumorigenic phenotype of SV_{40}-transformed cells remained unchanged at high doses of IFN, but appeared stimulated at low dosage. This latter result,

* In the course of these studies, we also cultivated the parental untransformed 10T1/2 cells in the continuous presence of IFN (Brouty-Boyé *et al.*, 1984). In the absence of IFN, spontaneous morphological transformation associated with increased saturation density could occur with extensive serial passage *in vitro*. These changes did not develop when untransformed 10T1/2 cells were passaged with IFN and they remained highly sensitive to IFN during the long-term treatment. These results suggest that IFN may also play a regulatory role in the maintenance of the integrity of the normal phenotype.

somewhat in conflict with the reduced ability of SV40-transformed cells to form colonies in agar *in vitro*, may again indicate a different regulatory role for IFN in cells transformed by different means. This is evident in the different refractory states that long-term treatment establishes in the three types of transformed cells. Thus, there was a decrease in the antiproliferative but not antiviral effects in IFN-treated x-ray-transformed cells that was reversible upon removal of IFN. In contrast, both effects were reduced in IFN-treated MCA-transformed cells although the level of 2-5A synthetase, which is thought to mediate one if not both effects, was induced to a high level. After several passages in the absence of IFN, MCA-transformed cells regained their initial sensitivity to the antiproliferative but not to the antiviral activity of IFN. No change of these types developed during long-term IFN treatment of SV_{40}-transformed cells.

The different responses to IFN exhibited by the same cell line transformed by three different agents clearly demonstrate the usefulness of cell systems of this type. They allow the characterization not only of the precise cellular functions essential to the maintenance of the tumour phenotype but also to those functions essential to the maintenance of the normal phenotype.

IFN-induced reversion has now been reported by others in several rodent cells transformed by different means. The data currently available are summarized in Table II. Positive results are obtained in cells transformed by different retroviruses (Moloney, Kirsten or Rous sarcoma viruses). It should be pointed out, however, that the degree of reversion induced by IFN in many of these systems cannot be fully estimated, since the parameters evaluated are mainly related to the transformed phenotype *in vitro*. Tumorigenicity tests need to be performed *in vivo* since reversal of transformed properties *in vitro* does not necessarily correlate with suppression of tumorigenicity. This is the case with MCA-transformed cells and more recently has been shown with murine Kirsten virus transformed cells, in which IFN reverses the transformed properties *in vitro* but surprisingly potentiates the tumorigenic phenotype (Wybier-Franqui, 1985). Reversion has also been shown to be induced in murine cells transformed by a human *ras* oncogene, whose transforming ability is due to its coupling to a retroviral activating sequence. On the other hand, transformation induced by a human *ras* gene, oncogenic because of a point mutation, is not reversed by IFN-treatment.

Morphological reversion and restoration of normal growth-related parameters has been found to occur in murine cells transformed by a bovine oncogenic DNA papilloma virus whose genome is present in a non-integrated form. In contrast, cells transformed by SV_{40} virus, which is integrated into the host DNA, do not revert when treated with IFN. In the case of non-viral-induced transformations, the best result is obtained in cells transformed by x-irradiation as opposed to chemically MCA-transformed cells. Since IFN

TABLE II Responses to IFN of Rodent Cells Transformed by Different Agents

Cells	Origin of oncogenicity	Oncogenic gene	Effects of IFN on[a]				Reference
			Transformed phenotype based on criteria of				
				Proliferation			
			Morphology	Liquid	Agar	Tumorigenic phenotype	
Transformed cells							
Murine	Virus	v-mos	+	+	+	+	Chany and Vignal (1970) Chany *et al.* (1985)
		v-Ki-ras[b]	+	+	+	ND	Hicks *et al.* (1981)
		v-Ki-ras	+	+	+	↑	Wybier-Franqui (1985)
		BPV_1-DNA[c]	+	+	+	ND	Tureck *et al.* (1982)
		SV_{40}-DNA[c]	–	+	+	↑	Brouty-Boyé *et al.* (1984)
	Human oncogenes	c-Ha-ras[d]	+	+	+	ND	Samid *et al.* (1983)
		c-Ha-ras[e]	–	ND	ND	ND	Samid *et al.* (1985)
	X-rays	?[f]	+	+	ND	+	Brouty-Boyé (1984)
	MCA	?	+	+	+	±	Brouty-Boyé *et al.* (1984)
Rat	Virus	v-Src[b]	+	+	ND	ND	Lin *et al.* (1983)
Murine tumour cells	MCA[b]	?	ND	+	ND	±	Wyvel and Pitha (1982)

[a] Cell response to IFN is scored as follows: change in cellular morphology (+); inhibition of cell proliferation (+); complete suppression of tumorigenicity (+); decreased rate of tumour growth and reduced number of mice with tumours (±); no change (–); potentiation of a given phenotypic parameter (↑).

[b] Phenotypic criteria evaluated after short-term IFN treatment.

[c] Bovine papilloma virus (BPV_1) DNA is not integrated in the host genome whereas SV_{40} is integrated.

[d] Cellular gene activated by the Ha-MuSV LTR and over-expression of a normal cellular protein.

[e] Gene activation resulting in the production of an altered cellular protein.

[f] Oncogene not yet identified.

ND = Not described.

reversed certain processes of induced transformation in rodent cells, the question of whether human IFN could induce similar changes in human tumour cells was investigated.

IV RESPONSES OF HUMAN TUMOUR CELLS TO LONG-TERM INTERFERON TREATMENT

The main source of human IFN in the past was that produced by Dr Kari Cantell's group, which for technical ease was prepared from human leucocytes. Although this natural IFN-α was not pure, it nevertheless proved to be effective in the treatment of several human diseases. The burst of interest in IFN research in the past few years led to improved techniques of production and purification of IFN from cell cultures and the cloning of certain species of human IFN-α. Since we did not know whether any individual recombinant species showed the same spectrum of activities as natural IFN-α, we chose to test initially the effects of purified IFN-α derived either from leucocytes (Mogensen and Cantell, 1977, 1979) or Namalva cells (Strander *et al.*, 1975). As regards the choice of tumour cells, we were inclined to test different human carcinoma cells, since over half of all primary cancer in man is from epithelial origin. Moreover, we also included tumour cells derived from osteosarcomas, because the first clinical trials with IFN initiated by Dr Hans Strander showed some efficacy against this type of malignancy (Strander *et al.*, 1973).

Tumour cell lines derived from two osteosarcomas, two urinary bladder carcinomas, one colon and one ovarian carcinoma were serially passaged in the continuous presence of 5,000 units of human IFN-α for extended periods of time*. The phenotype of the cells, based on criteria of proliferation, morphology, and tumorigenicity, was analysed at different passage levels.

The phenotypic changes induced by long-term IFN treatment differed markedly between the various tumour cells tested (Table III) (Brouty-Boyé *et al.*, 1985a). There was no drastic change in the morphology of the different tumour cell lines, with one exception, the G272 osteosarcoma cells, which exhibited large areas of epithelial-like morphology in the middle of sheets of elongated tumour cells (Fig. 2B). The changes, when they did occur, concerned principally the formation of cell piling or cell clumping (Fig. 2, Fig. 3). In some instances, even, opposite effects could be seen within the same cell lineage. For example, IFN suppressed cell piling in confluent cultures of

* Since the amount of IFN-α that inhibited the proliferation of human tumour cells was greater than that for transformed murine 10T1/2 cells, higher doses of human IFN were used.

Table III Different Responses of Human Tumour Cells to IFN

Cells	Oncogenic gene	Effects of IFN on[a]			
		Morphology	Cell clumping or cell aggregation	Proliferation	Tumorigenicity
Osteosarcoma					
G272	?	+	+	+	±
OHA	c-Ki-ras[b]	−	+	+	±
Carcinoma					
Colon	?	−	+	+	±
Bladder HT1376	?	−	+	+	−
Bladder EJ/T24	c-Ha-ras[b]	−	↑	+	↑
Ovary	?	−	−	+	±

[a] Score evaluation as in Table II.
[b] Gene activation resulting in the production of an altered cellular protein

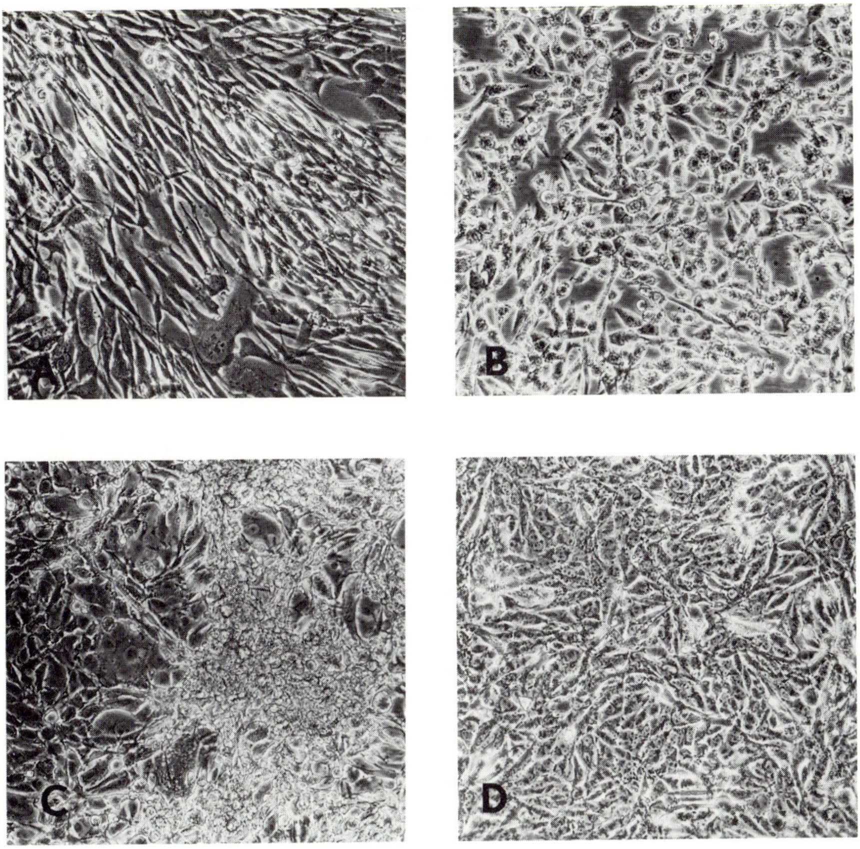

Fig. 2 Morphology of human osteosarcoma cells under long-term treatment with IFN-α. G272 tumour cells left untreated (**A**) or treated for 5 passages with IFN (**B**); OHA tumour cells left untreated (**C**) or treated for more than 10 passages with IFN (**D**).

one bladder tumour cell line (Fig. 3D) whereas more rounded dividing cells developed at confluency in the other cell line (Fig. 3F).

Inhibition of cellular proliferation was a consistent effect of IFN on all cell types tested. The degree of inhibition varied, however, from one cell type to another.

Less consistent results were obtained at the level of tumorigenicity (Table III). The tumorigenicity of osteosarcoma cells and colon carcinoma cells injected s.c. into nude mice was markedly reduced by passaging the cells with IFN. The reduction was evident by a reduced number of animals bearing tumours and a reduced rate of growth of the tumours. In contrast, bladder tumour cells treated with IFN remained tumorigenic and appeared

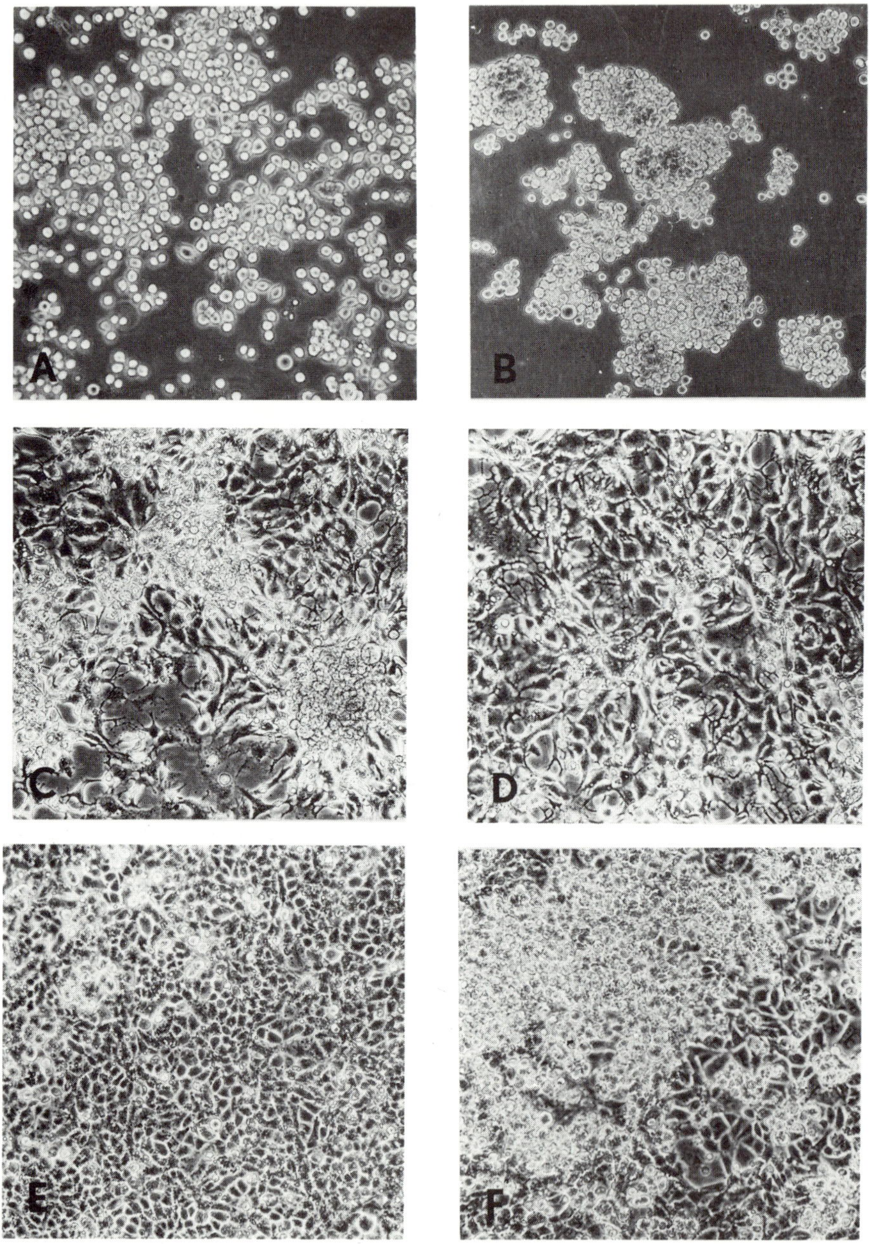

Fig. 3 Morphology of different human carcinoma cells under IFN-α treatment. Colon carcinoma C0205 cells left untreated (**A**) or treated for 5 passages with IFN-α (**B**); bladder carcinoma HT1376 cells left untreated (**C**) or treated for 10 passages with IFN-α (**D**); bladder carcinoma EJ/T24 cells left untreated (**E**) or treated for more than 10 passages with IFN-α (**F**).

even more tumorigenic than untreated cells, while the tumorigenicity of IFN-treated ovarian tumour cells was slightly reduced when injected i.p. but not when injected s.c.

It is important to mention here that the phenotypic effects described above occurred more or less progressively within the first 10 passages. When two of these tumour cell lines were maintained with IFN for more extended periods of time, the IFN-induced changes in the tumour cell phenotype persisted for one cell line (osteosarcoma cells) whereas for another cell line (colon tumour cells) they decreased.

In summary, our results show that IFN alters the phenotype of human tumour cells in diverse ways. However, in no instance did these changes result in a full reversal of the human tumour cell phenotype (that is, complete suppression of tumorigenicity). At best, there was partial reversion for some IFN-treated cell lines. These findings emphasize the need for a greater characterization and understanding of the variables and mechanisms that may account for the differences in the cell response to IFN.

V VARIABLES THAT MAY INFLUENCE THE HETEROGENEOUS RESPONSE TO INTERFERON

Preliminary experiments that yielded only a partial estimation of the numerous variables that may influence the cell response to IFN showed that clones derived from a colon carcinoma cell line differed in their sensitivity to the antiproliferative activity of IFN-α. The tumorigenic phenotype of the most sensitive clone was significantly more reduced by IFN treatment than that of parental tumour cells. Thus, the degree of heterogeneity of the tumour cell population appears to be important.

It seems that the phenotypic effects of IFN varied according to the species of IFN used. Thus, inhibition of cell proliferation, enhancement in cell aggregation and reduction in tumorigenicity of colon carcinoma cells were more pronounced when the cells were continuously exposed to IFN-γ than when treated with IFN-α (Brouty-Boyé, unpublished observations).

Environmental conditions *in vitro* also appear to play an important role in the expression of particular phenotypic changes. Thus, aggregation of IFN-treated colon cells was not observed when these cells were seeded on collagen-coated plastic instead of bare plastic, or when cultivated in calcium-free medium (Brouty-Boyé *et al.*, 1985a). Moreover, the partial reversion of the tumorigenic phenotype induced by IFN-γ in colon carcinoma cells was totally abrogated by serial passages of IFN-treated cells on "extracellular matrices" (Wybier-Franqui and Brouty-Boyé, unpublished observations). Even *in vivo*, we found that the tumorigenic phenotype of IFN-treated ovarian cells was reduced when the cells were injected i.p., but barely affected when the cells were injected s.c.

An even more fundamental variable may be at the level of *the processes implicated in tumorigenesis*. It is now evident that malignant transformation is triggered by distinct primary oncogenic events. Indeed, oncogenic transformation can be initiated either by the introduction into the cells of an active transforming gene as a result of infection by DNA tumour viruses or by the conversion of a small set of cellular genes, normally silent, into transforming genes when activated inappropriately by the cells, retrovirus infection and possibly exposure to various kinds of radiations and chemicals. Consequently, there is either production of new specific proteins derived from the activity of the viral genome, or production of an altered cellular protein, or overproduction of a normal protein resulting from activated cellular genes. By interacting with one or multiple cellular sites, these distinct oncogenic products are thought to be responsible for the many cellular changes that accompany oncogenic transformation.

It is conceivable that the IFN-induced reversion occurred because of an interaction at any one of the steps in this complex chain of events. The first possibility concerns effects implicated in the pathway leading to oncogenic protein production. Indeed, some data demonstrate an association between IFN-induced reversion and disappearance of viral transforming DNA* (Tureck *et al.*, 1982); reduction in mRNAs of certain cellular oncogenes (Samid *et al.*, 1984); and reduction in transforming gene products (Lin *et al.*, 1983). Furthermore, although there seems to be no relation between the activation of viruses and the transformation process induced by x-irradiation, we found in one of the two clones tested the presence of C-type viral particles. In this case, IFN decreased the viral expression along with the reversion of the transformed and tumorigenic phenotype (Brouty-Boyé and Gresser, 1981). From recent findings obtained in human tumour cells, it appears, however, that changes in oncogenic pathways is not a prerequisite for IFN-induced reversion.

As described above, our investigations of the effects of IFN on the phenotype of human tumour cells showed that a long-term treatment with IFN induced a partial reversion in tumour cells derived from an osteosarcoma. This was evident by a marked reduction in cell proliferation, lack of cellular overlapping in confluent culture, and a significant reduction in tumorigenicity.

* It should be noted that this result concerns a non-integrated oncogenic DNA virus. When the cells were transformed by the integrated SV_{40} virus, the viral genome persisted, as evidenced by the presence of the T antigen in IFN-treated cells, and no reversion was induced (Brouty-Boyé *et al.*, 1984).

Nevertheless, the transforming ability, genomic level and expression of the *c-Ki-ras* oncogene activated in these tumour cells were not modified by IFN-treatment (Brouty-Boyé *et al.*, 1985b). More recently, it has been found that in IFN-treated murine MSV-transformed fibroblasts, the genomic level of the viral transforming v-mos sequence was increased despite the reversal of the transformed phenotype (Chany *et al.*, 1985). These data suggest that, instead of directly acting on oncogenic pathways, IFN can affect the phenotype of certain tumour cells by altering the cell response to oncogene products.

Evidence has accumulated that indicates that IFN regulates the expression of several cellular proteins (Friedman *et al.*, 1984). Although little is known about the exact functions of most of these proteins, we can surmise that they may be part of those essential cellular proteins that are responsible for the maintenance of the normal phenotype. They would, therefore, render oncogenic products unable, by themselves, to maintain malignant properties.

VI IS INTERFERON-INDUCED REVERSION A PLAUSIBLE MECHANISM FOR THE ANTITUMOUR ACTIVITY OF INTERFERON?

Total and partial regression of a certain number of solid tumours has been observed in man under IFN treatment (Borden, 1983). Whether these regressions are attributable to changes in tumour cell phenotype or to other causes remains an unanswered question. There are, however, some examples which by their similarities to systems *in vitro* suggest that reversion may be implicated. A therapeutic success has been obtained in the treatment of human juvenile laryngeal papilloma that is acknowledged to be of viral etiology (Haglund *et al.*, 1981). Since it has been demonstrated *in vitro* that reversion is observed under long-term treatment of mouse cells transformed by a bovine papilloma virus in association with a disappearance in viral transforming DNA (Tureck *et al.*, 1982), it is possible that regression of these tumours *in vivo* has occurred through similar mechanisms.

Another example that may illustrate the conversion of tumour cells into cells that have lost their malignant properties is that of hairy-cell leukemia, a B-cell neoplam. Similar to reversion *in vitro*, which is induced by long-term IFN treatment, long-term IFN therapy is required to achieve complete remission in patients with hairy-cell leukemia (Quesada *et al.*, 1984).

It is clearly of practical importance to demonstrate IFN-induced reversion *in vivo*. To date, there is no experimental evidence. The difficulty may reside in the choice of appropriate experimental systems and/or in the choice of criteria to assess reversion.

In the attempts to determine whether IFN could induce reversion *in vivo*, experimental models were used that retained potentialities for expressing programmes of differentiation.

Employing the murine Friend leukemic cells, it has recently been shown that IFN treatment induced the complete regression of these tumours (Belardelli *et al.*, 1982, 1983). There was, however, no evidence of cellular differentiation (Belardelli *et al.*, 1982) even though IFN caused these cells to differentiate *in vitro* (Cioè *et al.*, 1978). Similar results were obtained in testing myeloma cells (Vignaux *et al.*, 1984) or teratocarcinoma cells (Gresser *et al.*, 1984) in mice.

These studies would suggest that IFN-treated tumour cells might not have to attain, *in vivo*, the terminal stage of differentiation to lose their malignant properties. Reappearance of markers of the differentiated phenotype would then not be appropriate criteria. Another possibility is that the reversal of malignant phenotype might not necessarily mean the return to a truly "normal" cell. In fact, from our studies on x-ray transformed cells, it is apparent that IFN-reverted cells differed in several respects from parental untransformed cells although they displayed many of the characteristics of normal cells. Their morphology was not quite similar and their sensitivity to IFN remained low. Even though IFN-reverted cells were not exactly like normal cells, they were nevertheless, unable to proliferate in animals. They, therefore, fulfilled the ultimate criteria for reversion.

VII CLOSING REMARKS

Studies on the long-term effects of IFN on transformed and tumour cells in culture allowed us to distinguish two types of effects that differ in the timing of their expression: short-term effects expressed within a few days, and effects only observed after prolonged treatment. That these long-term effects are secondary to early events is possible, but they require the continuous presence of IFN. Short-term effects, however, can decline despite further incubation of the cells with IFN. Removal of IFN usually restores the initial level of sensitivity in the cells.

It seems likely that more than one effect of IFN is responsible for the reversal of the tumour cell phenotype. Several examples indicate that IFN-induced changes in some parameters of transformation are not sufficient by themselves to convert fully a tumour cell into a normal cell. IFN might succeed in inducing complete reversion in a stepwise fashion.

It is evident that IFN can redirect tumour cells towards a normal stage by acting at different levels: viral replication, oncogenic protein production, and the cellular response to the action of the oncogenic products. However, the action of IFN appears to be bidirectional. Although in many cells IFN reverses some or all of the characteristics associated with malignancy, in some instances IFN potentiates the phenotypic characteristics of transformed and tumour cells. By the nature of the diversity of the malignant processes which appear to include distinct oncogenic products and cellular targets, it seems rather unlikely that IFN should affect these processes in the same way. Characterizing the mechanisms involved in the bidirectional action of IFN should lead to a better understanding of the emergence or loss of malignancy.

If reversion can be induced *in vivo*, the therapy of cancer might be directed to the use of substances capable of reversing the neoplastic state. On the basis of data *in vitro*, it appears that in some situations IFN can induce reversion while in other instances it fails to induce reversion. It is conceivable that, if used in combination with other compounds that can also induce reversion, IFN therapy would be more efficient in the control of tumour growth *in vivo*.

ACKNOWLEDGEMENTS

I am grateful to Dr Ion Gresser for his leadership and enthusiasm in investigating new areas of IFN research. His pioneering contributions to the non-antiviral effects of IFN have encouraged numerous investigations leading to the discovery of a wide variety of different regulatory functions for IFN. I thank the following for their skilful collaboration, critical comments and encouragement, which have brought these long-term studies to their current status: M-T. Bandu, C. Calvo, T. Lampidis, C. Maury, K. E. Mogensen, H. Suarez, F. Vignaux, J. Wybier-Franqui, F. Zambetti. This work was supported in part by grants from the Institut National de la Santé et de la Recherche Médicale, the Association pour la Recherche sur le Cancer à Villejuif, the Richard Lounsbery Foundation and the Direction des Recherches, Etudes et Technique (contract 82–420).

REFERENCES

Aguet, M. (1980). *Nature* (*London*) **284**, 459–461.

Belardelli, F., Gresser, I., Maury, C. and Maunoury, M. T. (1982). *Int. J. Cancer* **30**, 813–820.

Belardelli, F., Gresser, I., Maury, C., Duvillard, P., Prade, M. and Maunoury M. T. (1983). *Int. J. Cancer* **31**, 649–653.

Borden, E. C. (1983). *In* "Interferon 83" (I. Gresser, ed.), vol. 5, pp. 43–83. Academic Press, New York.

Brouty-Boyé, D. (1980). *Lymphokine Rep.* **1**, 99–112.

Brouty-Boyé, D. (1982). *Int. J. Cancer* **30**, 193–195.

Brouty-Boyé, D. and Gresser, I. (1981). *Int. J. Cancer* **28**, 165–173.
Brouty-Boyé, D., Gresser, I. and Baldwin, C. (1979). *Int. J. Cancer* **24**, 253–260.
Brouty-Boyé, D., Cheng, Y. E. and Chen, L. B. (1981). *Cancer Res.* **41**, 4174–4184.
Brouty-Boyé, D., Gresser, I. and Bandu, M. T. (1982a). *Carcinogenesis* **9**, 1057–1061.
Brouty-Boyé, D., Puvion-Dutilleul, F. and Gresser, I. (1982b). *Experientia* **38**, 1292–1296.
Brouty-Boyé, D., Wybier-Franqui, J., Calvo, C., Feunteun, J. and Gresser, I. (1984). *Int. J. Cancer* **34**, 107–112.
Brouty-Boyé, D., Mogensen, K. E. and Gresser, I. (1985a). *Eur. J. Cancer Clin. Oncol.* **21**, 507–514.
Brouty-Boyé, D., Wybier-Franqui, J., Suarez, H. and Gresser, I. (1985b). *In* "The Interferon System" (F. Dianzani and G. B. Rossi, eds.), vol 24, pp. 303–307. Raven Press, New York.
Chany, C. and Vignal, M. (1970). *J. Gen. Virol.* **7**, 203–210.
Chany, C., Gerfeaux, J. and Sergiescu, D. (1985). TNO-ISIR Meeting on the Interferon System, Clearwater Beach, Florida, p. 33 (abstract).
Cioè, L., Dolei, A., Rossi, G. B., Belardelli, F., Affabris, E., Gambari, E. and Fantoni, A. (1978). *In* "In Vitro Aspects of Erythropoeisis" (M. Murphy, ed.), pp. 159–171. Springer-Verlag, Berlin and New York.
De Maeyer-Guignard, J., Tovey, M. G., Gresser, I. and De Maeyer, E. (1978). *Nature (London)* **271**, 622–625.
Friedman, R. L., Mauly, S. P., McMahon, M., Kerr, I. M. and Stark, G. R. (1984). *Cell* **38**, 745–755.
Gresser, I. (1961). *Proc. Natl Acad. Sci. USA* **47**, 1817–1822.
Gresser, I. (1977). *In* "Cancer a Comprehensive Treatrise" (F. Becker, ed.), vol. 5, pp. 521–571. Plenum Press, New York.
Gresser, I., Coppey, J., Fontaine-Brouty-Boyé, D., Falcoff, R., Falcoff, E. and Zajdela, F. (1967). *Nature (London)* **215**, 174–175.
Gresser, I., Maury, C., Bandu, M. T., Foiret, D., Trojan, J. and Uriel, J. (1984). *J. Interferon Res.* **4**, 375–381.
Haglund, S., Lundquist, P. G., Cantell, K. and Strander, H. (1981). *Arch. Otolaryngol* **107**, 327–332.
Hicks, N. J., Morris, A. G. and Burke, D. C. (1981). *J. Cell. Sci.* **49**, 225–236.
Lin, S. L., Garber, E. A., Wang, E., Caliguir, L. A., Schellekens, H., Goldberg, A. R. and Tamm, I. (1983). *Mol. Cell. Biol.* **3**, 1656–1664.
Mintz, B. and Illmensee, K. (1975). *Proc. Natl Acad. Sci. USA* **72**, 3585–3589.
Mogensen, K. E. and Cantell, K. (1977). *Pharmacol. Ther. (C)* **1**, 369–381.
Mogensen, K. E. and Cantell, K. (1979). *J. Gen. Virol.* **45**, 171–175.
Oxman, M. N., Baron, S., Black, P. H., Takimok, K., Habel, K. and Rowe, W. P. (1967). *Virology* **32**, 122–127.
Quesada, J. R., Reuben, J., Manning, J. T., Hersh, E. M. and Gutterman, J. U. (1984). *New Engl. J. Med.* **310**, 15–18.
Samid, D., Chang, E. H. and Friedman, R. M. (1984). *Biochem. Biophys. Res. Commun.* **119**, 21–28.
Samid, D., Chang, E. H. and Friedman, R. M. (1985). *Biochem. Biophys. Res. Commun.* **126**, 509–516.
Strander, H., Cantell, K., Carlström, G. and Jacobsson, P. A. (1973). *J. Natl Cancer Inst.* **51**, 733–735.
Taylor-Papadimitriou, J. (1982). *In* "Interferon 1980" (I. Gresser, ed.) vol. 2, pp. 13–46. Academic Press, New York.

Topp, W. C., Lane, D. and Pollack, R. (1980). *In* "DNA Tumour Viruses, Molecular Biology of Tumor Viruses" (J. Tooze, ed.), pp. 205–296. Cold Spring Harbor Laboratory Publications.

Tovey, M. G., Begon-Lours, J. and Gresser, I. (1974). *Proc. Soc. Exp. Biol. Med.* **146**, 809–815.

Tureck, L. P., Byrne, J. C., Lowy, D. R., Dvoretzky, I., Friedman, R. M. and Howley, P. M. (1982). *Proc. Natl Acad. Sci. USA* **79**, 7914–7918.

Vignaux, F., Stanislawski, M. and Gresser, I. (1983). *Ann. Immunol. Inst. Pasteur* **135**. 187–194.

Wyblier-Franqui, J. (1985). Ares-Serono Symposium on the Interferon System, Rome, May 8–11, p. 124 (abstract).

Wyvel, N. A. and Pitha, P. M. (1982). *Int. J. Cancer* **30**, 649–654.

Interferons and the Regulation of Oncogenes

GERALD J. JONAK AND ERNEST KNIGHT, Jr

E. I. du Pont de Nemours and Co. Inc., Central Research and Development Department, Wilmington, Delaware 19898 USA

I INTRODUCTION

What do interferons (IFNs) and oncogenes have in common? Both have been implicated in the regulation of cellular functions. As early as 1962 Paucker, Cantell, and Henle reported that preparations of interferon inhibited the growth of cells in culture. These initial observations on the anti-proliferative activity of IFN were followed by findings that IFN prevented a DNA tumour virus-induced cellular transformation (Todaro and Green, 1967), and that prolonged IFN treatment induced phenotypic reversion in murine sarcoma virus-transformed mouse fibroblasts (Chany and Vignal, 1970). As documented by a number of excellent review articles in this series and elsewhere, these important observations have been confirmed and extended in other experimental systems, all suggesting that IFN is an important natural growth and cell function modifier.

Nearly two decades later, cellular genes called oncogenes have been implicated in the regulation of cell growth, development, differentiation, and

INTERFERON 7
ISBN 0 12 302256 8

the capacity to transform normal cells into neoplastic cancer cells (see below). The intensive and broad research in the oncogene area has generated a considerable body of knowledge having important implications for our understanding of the regulation of cellular genes and genesis of neoplasia. Because of the wealth of related information in both areas, it therefore appears self-evident to ask the simple question (undoubtedly followed by arrays of complex answers) whether IFN has the capacity to regulate qualitatively or quantitatively specific oncogenes and whether this may be related to some aspects of its biological activity. Furthermore, this type of study may aid in our understanding of how IFN regulates the expression and function of cellular genes in general. In this article we review reports in which mRNA or protein products of oncogenes have been analysed after the treatment of cells with IFN.

This article reviews only the effects of IFN on cellular and not viral oncogenes, since an excellent review on that and related topics appeared recently (Clemens and McNurlan, 1985). The reader should be aware that all publications in this area have appeared in the last two years and it is very likely that the interpretation of current data may change in the future. However, we feel that as in other aspects of real life, the relationship of the mature and vigorous (interferon field) with the young and attractive (oncogene field) may prove beneficial to both.

II CELLULAR ONCOGENES

One of the fundamental discoveries of the last decade has been the finding that normal cells harbour genes that share sequence homology with the oncogenes of acutely transforming RNA tumour viruses (v-*onc*) and/or have the capacity to confer the transformed phenotype on normal cells in transfection assays (reviewed by Bishop 1983, Cooper and Lane, 1984, Weinberg 1985). Transfection assays measure the ability of DNA (from tumour cells or cloned genes) to induce morphologically transformed foci on a background of non-transformed cells such as the immortalized NIH 3T3 fibroblasts or primary cells (Shih *et al.*, 1979; Land *et al.*, 1983). Transforming capacity can be further assayed by growth of transfectants in semisolid medium (Cooper *et al.*, 1980) or by their capacity to form tumours in nude mice (Blair *et al.*, 1982). Because of such attributes, these resident cellular genes have been termed cellular oncogenes (c-*onc*).*

*The c-*onc*, identified in DNA from tumour cells by transfection assays, have also been termed "transforming genes" or "tumour genes". The cellular progenitors of v-*onc* or any cellular gene with the potential of becoming an oncogene are sometimes referred to as 'proto-oncogenes". For the sake of brevity, we have elected to use the term cellular oncogenes for all these genes. An interested and critical reader should consult the above review articles, which cover the subject in more detail. Also, for an alternative view on the role and function of cellular oncogenes, the articles of Duesberg (1983, 1985) are of interest.

The c-*onc* have been detected in species as disparate as human, rodent, avian, and also in worms, *Drosophila* and yeast (Bishop 1981; Shilo and Weinberg 1981; DeFeo-Jones et al., 1983). In normal cells and tissues they are expressed and regulated in a cell cycle, developmental or differentiation-specific manner (Kelly *et al.*, 1983; Verma *et al.*, 1984). The evolutionary conservation and regulatable expression in normal cells implies that these cellular genes are required for essential metabolic functions and integrity of eukaryotic cells. Only when activated (misregulated or structurally altered), does their expression in cells redound to neoplasia and cancer. Several mechanisms may lead to the process of c-*onc* activation. The most notable one is the generation of the v-*onc* themselves. The v-*onc* have been transduced into RNA tumour viruses (retroviruses) by a recombination event between one or even two c-*onc* mRNAs and a retroviral genome. A number of c-*onc* are therefore progenitors of v-*onc* (evidence reviewed by Bishop 1983). During this process, not only are c-*onc* coding sequences often altered, but they become regulated by viral control elements, and thus are expressed independently of the original cellular regulation. Structural analysis of c-*onc* in tumour cells has led to the discovery of additional activation mechanisms. They include: structural mutations in the c-*onc* coding regions (Capon *et al.*, 1983; Taparowsky *et al.*, 1983), c-*onc* gene amplification (Collins and Groudine, 1982), translocation of c-*onc* to different chromosomal locations (Taub *et al.*, 1982), and integration of viral regulatory elements in the vicinity of c-*onc* (Hayward *et al.*, 1981). The c-*onc* activated by these processes would either produce protein products that are functionally different from its normal counterparts, or no longer be subject to stringent cellular regulations required for controlled growth of normal cells and tissues.

Structural and functional homologies have been noted between three oncogenic proteins and cellular growth control elements: the *sis* oncogene encodes a protein similar to the platelet-derived growth factor (Waterfield *et al.*, 1983), *erb*-B is a truncated form of the epidermal growth factor receptor (Downward *et al.*, 1984) and the product of the *ras* family of oncogenes is analogous to the intracellular G proteins that transduce signals from cell-surface hormone receptors to adenyl cyclase (McGrath *et al.*, 1984). The expression of these oncogenes in cells would allow their escape from the dependence on exogenous growth signals and regulation by an autocrine mechanism (*sis*), a receptor modification (*erb*-B) or a transducer alteration (*ras*). Even though this is at best an over-simplified scenario, this type of structural analysis and functional comparison of oncogenic proteins with their normal counterparts will be instrumental for our understanding of the role of oncogenes in growth control (Weinberg, 1985).

Another important question, however, concerns the mechanisms by which normal cells regulate the expression and functions of c-*onc* and whether tumour cells are still capable of such regulation, especially when they harbour activated oncogenes. Investigations into the mechanism by which IFN exerts its growth modulatory activity in normal and tumour cells may provide us with important insights on the regulation of cellular oncogenes.

III CELLULAR ONCOGENES AND THE EFFECT OF INTERFERONS

A c-*fos*

The v-*fos* oncogene of the Finkel-Biskis-Jinkins murine osteosarcoma virus has cellular homologues (c-*fos*) in the genome of various vertebrates, including human and mouse (Curran *et al.*, 1982). The genomic c-*fos* does not transform cells, but the addition of a transcriptional enhancer and the disruption of the 3′ end of the gene activates its transforming potential (Miller *et al.*, 1984). Expression of c-*fos* mRNA and protein (located in the nucleus) has been detected during prenatal and postnatal development in humans and mice (Müller *et al.*, 1984a; Verma *et al.*, 1984). Expression of either human or mouse c-*fos* in transfected F9 mouse teratocarcinoma cells resulted in differentiation-like morphological changes accompanied by the appearance of several markers characteristic of trophoblastic and endodermal cells (Müller and Wagner, 1984). A rapid but transient c-*fos* induction (transcription, mRNA and protein) appeared as a part of the competence process in quiescent mouse 3T3 cells stimulated with growth factors (Greenberg and Ziff, 1984; Müller *et al.*, 1984b). In addition to its transforming capacity, c-*fos* may therefore also play a role in development, differentiation, and regulation of cell growth.

The effect on c-*fos* mRNA expression and its relationship to the inhibition of cell growth by IFN (α and β) has been analysed by Einat *et al.*, (1985a). The authors observed that the increase in c-*fos* mRNA that occurred within 20 minutes in quiescent Balb/c 3T3 cells upon the addition of either serum or platelet-derived growth factor (PDGF) had been reduced by 50–80% following concomitant exposure of the cells to 100 units/ml of mouse IFN. The mitogenic response of such treated cells was also significantly inhibited. The IFN did not, however, simply interfere with the binding of PDGF to its receptors, as the PDGF-mediated increase in the uptake of deoxyglucose was unimpaired by the IFN treatment. In addition to the reduction of c-*fos*, a reduction in the level of the mRNAs of β-actin, ornithine decarboxylase and c-*myc* (see below) was also observed. These genes, whose expression is induced in quiescent cells by PDGF, are believed to be a part of the regulatory mechanism that makes cells competent to progress from G_0 to G_1.

Since the inhibition of cell growth by IFN occurs primarily during the G_1 transition, the authors speculated that the anti-proliferative effect of IFN may, at least in part, be mediated through the repression of competence genes. A delicate balance between the induction and repression of the competence genes, including c-*fos*, mediated by PDGF and IFN would therefore determine the proliferative state of the cells. This notion may explain the previously published results describing the reversal of the anti-mitogenic effect of IFN by an excess of PDGF (Inglot *et al.*, 1980).

B c-*myc*

The avian, human and mouse c-*myc* genes are the cellular homologues of the avian myelocytomatosis virus (MC29) oncogene, v-*myc*. The expression of c-*myc* mRNA and proteins has been detected in a wide spectrum of normal cells and tissues. While the c-*myc* expression (mRNA and protein) is relatively constant in different stages of the cell cycle in proliferating cells (Hann *et al.*, 1985; Thompson *et al.*, 1985), it is very low, or below detection levels, in non-proliferating cells (Kelly *et al.*, 1983; Müller *et al.*, 1984b). A rapid, many-fold induction of c-*myc* mRNA occurs within 2–3 hours following stimulation of non-proliferating cells (fibroblasts, lymphocytes) with cell-specific mitogens or growth-promoting agents (see review by Kelly and Siebenlist, 1985). On the other hand, the c-*myc* expression is rapidly inhibited in cells whose proliferation ceased as the result of differentiation events (Reitsma *et al.*, 1983; Dony *et al.*, 1985; Einat *et al.*, 1985b). One of the functions of c-*myc* in normal cells (like the c-*fos*, see above), may therefore be in the regulation of cell proliferation.

As mentioned above in connection with c-*fos*, Einat *et al.* (1985a) have shown that IFN (α and β) inhibited the PDGF-mediated stimulation of c-*myc* mRNA in Balb/c 3T3 cells. The inhibition of c-*myc* mRNA was more pronounced than the c-*fos*, measuring 95% after 3 hours. The inhibition was much less evident in the presence of cycloheximide, indicating that the IFN-mediated mechanism regulating c-*myc* mRNA depends on either new or sustained protein synthesis. As with the c-*fos*, the authors speculated that the c-*myc* repression may be related to the anti-proliferative effect of IFN in this system.

The c-*myc* expression is also believed to play a role in the process of neoplastic transformation. While c-*myc* alone is not transforming, it will, in combination with the *ras* oncogene, transform primary cells as determined by their immortalized *in vitro* phenotype and tumour formation in nude mice (Land *et al.*, 1983). Structural features of c-*myc* are often altered in avian, human and mouse tumour cells. Insertions of viral transcriptional regulatory sequences in the vicinity of the c-*myc* gene have been detected in avian B cell lymphomas (Hayward *et al.*, 1981) and murine T-cell leukemias (Corcoran *et al.*, 1984). Chromosomal aberations, involving the translocation of the c-*myc* gene into chromosomal segments harbouring immunoglobulin genes, occur specifically in mouse plasmacytomas and Burkitt lymphomas (Taub *et al.*, 1982; Shen-Ong *et al.*, 1982). The c-*myc* oncogene is amplified in the human promyelocytic cell line HL-60 (Collins and Groudine, 1982). Such structural alterations together with mutations and/or rearrangements that often occur within the c-*myc* gene activate its expression, thus resulting in unregulated proliferation and the genesis of neoplasia.

In the Burkitt lymphoma cell line Daudi, whose growth is inhibited by low levels of IFN-α or -β, the c-*myc* mRNA was found to be consistently reduced by more than 75% after IFN treatment (Jonak and Knight, 1984; Dani *et al.*, 1985; Einat *et al.*, 1985b). These results are of interest, as they show that the IFNs have the capacity to repress the expression of the c-*myc* oncogene that is activated in these cells by translocation of the gene from chromosome 8 to 14. The reduction in the steady-state level of c-*myc* mRNA was detectable as early as 1 hour after the addition of IFN-β, and appears to be mediated by a post-transcriptional mechanism, since the transcription of the c-*myc* gene was unaffected even after 24 hours of IFN-β treatment (Dani *et al.*, 1985; Knight *et al.*, 1985a). IFN-induced protein synthesis was not required as the reduction occurred even in the presence of cycloheximide (Knight *et al.*, 1985b). Furthermore, a 67–80% reduction in the half-life of c-*myc* mRNA has been detected in these cells following IFN-treatment (Dani *et al.*, 1985). Another report, however, showed that IFN inhibited the c-*myc* gene transcription, and that the c-*myc* mRNA half-life was reduced only slightly (Einat *et al.*, 1985b; Kimchi *et al.*, 1985a, b). These disparate results may either reflect diverse regulatory mechanisms in variant Daudi cell lines, or be due to methodological variables such as the use of different c-*myc* probes.

The c-*myc* mRNA reduction in Daudi cells precedes the IFN-mediated inhibition of cell growth by several hours, indicating that it is not merely a consequence of cessation of cell growth. Furthermore, in Daudi cell variants (Dron and Tovey, 1983) and several Burkitt cell lines (Namalva, Raji, Manca, BL67) that are resistant to the anti-proliferative activity of IFN, the c-*myc* mRNA is not reduced (Einat *et al.* 1985b; Jonak *et al.*, 1985a; Knight *et al.*, 1985b; Salehzada *et al.*, 1985; Dron *et al.*, 1985). Based on these results, the above groups speculated that a reduced expression of c-*myc* mRNA may play a role in the inhibition of cell growth by IFN. However, the correlation between the c-*myc* mRNA reduction and the IFN-mediated inhibition of cell growth is not always evident. The steady-state level of c-*myc* mRNA was not reduced, but slightly increased in PDGF-induced Balb/c 3T3 cells pretreated for 48 hours with mouse IFN-β. The proliferative response of these cells was nevertheless inhibited (Tominaga and Lengyel, 1985). In proliferating HeLa cells, IFN-α reduced the c-*myc* mRNA level by 50% within 4 hours of exposure, while IFN-γ, even though profoundly inhibiting HeLa cell growth, actually stimulated the c-*myc* mRNA 3-fold (Kelly *et al.*, 1985). In Daudi cells that reverted to IFN sensitivity from an IFN-resistant phenotype, the inhibition of cell growth was not preceded by a significant reduction in the c-*myc* mRNA (Knight *et al.* 1985b; Dron *et al.*, 1985). In these revertant cells, a reduction in the c-*myc* mRNA occurred only after 24–48 hours of IFN-treatment. However, after that period of IFN exposure, the mRNA level of other cellular genes, e.g. actin, was also reduced, suggesting a generalized decline in cellular mRNAs. These results indicate that if a functional connection between the expression and/or function of c-*myc* and the IFN-mediated inhibition of cell growth existed, it would have to involve more than a reduction in the level of c-*myc* mRNA.

Proteins presumed to be c-*myc*-specific have been immunoprecipitated with antisera raised against either synthetic peptides or "c-*myc*-like" proteins expressed in bacteria. Proteins with molecular weights ranging from 62,000 to 68,000 have been reported for a variety of human cells (Hann and Eisenman, 1984; Ramsay *et al.*, 1984; Persson *et al.*, 1984). The c-*myc* proteins appear to be localized in the nucleus (Hann and Eisenman, 1984; Persson and Leder, 1984) and may function as intracellular mediators of mitogenesis. In support of this notion, it has been shown that either a transfected c-*myc* gene or microinjected c-*myc* protein can partially replace the growth requirement for PDGF in mouse 3T3 cells (Armelin *et al.*, 1984; Kaczmarek *et al.*, 1985). In our laboratory we have shown that IFN treatment of sensitive Daudi cells causes a decrease in the synthesis of the two c-*myc* proteins of 66,000 and 63,000 daltons while causing an appearance of a new protein of 61,000 daltons (Knight and Jonak, unpublished observations). The 61,000-dalton protein might be derived by either altered processing of the 63,000- or 66,000-dalton proteins; or it might be a protein induced by IFN, structurally unrelated to the c-*myc* protein(s), but immunoprecipitated because of a tight association with the c-*myc* protein(s). All of these proteins were immunoprecipitated by antisera raised to synthetic peptides whose amino acid sequence corresponds to a region near either the *C*- or *N*-terminus of the predicted c-*myc* protein. It will be of interest to determine the c-*myc* protein level in cells whose growth is inhibited by IFN but for which the steady-state level of c-*myc* mRNA is not reduced. These results would provide additional information on whether the reduction of c-*myc* expression by IFN treatment plays a role in growth cessation.

C c-*ras*^{H}

The transforming oncogenes in about 20% of human tumour DNAs scoring positive in the NIH/3T3 transfection assay are cellular homologues of either the Harvey (v-*ras*^{H}) or Kirsten (v-*ras*^{K}) sarcoma virus oncogenes (Cooper and Lane, 1984). The protein product of the c-*ras* oncogenes has a molecular weight of approximately 21,000 daltons and is known as p21. Microinjection of either mouse or human p21, made in *E. coli*, into quiescent mouse 3T3 cells resulted in loss of growth control, as evidenced by the induction of DNA synthesis, cell division, and the appearance of transformed morphology (Feramisco *et al.*, 1984; Stacey and Kung, 1984). The p21 is localized on the inner surface of the plasma membrane, binds and hydrolyses guanosine triphosphate, and has autophosphorylating activity (McGrath *et al.*, 1984; Gibbs *et al.*, 1984). Functional and structural similarities have been noted between the p21 and the guanine nucleotide-binding proteins that regulate the adenylate cyclase activity following the binding of hormones to their membrane receptors (McGrath *et al.*, 1984). The transforming potential of the c-*ras*^{H} and c-*ras*^{K} is activated by either over-expression of normal p21 or structural mutations altering amino acids in or around positions 12 or 61 in the p21 protein (Chang *et al.*, 1982; Capon *et al.*, 1983). The p21, either in its normal or activated form, may therefore regulate cellular growth and phenotype by influencing the level of adenyl cyclase activity.

Several experimental models have been employed to study the effect of IFN on the expression of either endogenous or transfected c-*ras* oncogenes. Treatment of human bladder carcinoma cells (RT4) with human IFN-β resulted in a reduced mRNA expression from the resident c-*ras*^{H}, but not c-*ras*^{K} oncogenes (Soslau *et al.*, 1984). The reduction appeared to be related to the cessation of the tumour cell growth, as it was evident only in cells treated with doses of IFN-β inducing both the antiviral and antiproliferative response, and occurred prior to changes in their growth rate. These authors also reported that IFN-β altered the phosphorylation of a protein of approximately 21,000 daltons and suggested that it might be the product of the p21 gene, but presented no further supporting evidence. A reduced level of c-*ras*^{H} mRNA has also been detected in IFN-β treated NIH 3T3 mouse cells transformed with a cloned human c-*ras*^{H}, activated by the transcriptional control elements of Harvey sarcoma virus (Samid *et al.*, 1984). In these cells, grown for 20–40 generations with IFN, the reduction was correlated with the appearance of revertant, non-transformed cells characterized by contact inhibition, low saturation density, inability to grow in soft agar and failure to produce tumours in nude mice. While the structure and copy number of the transforming c-*ras*^{H} oncogene was unchanged in these revertants, the rate of its transcription was reduced and this may account for the observed reduction in steady-state level of c-*ras*^{H} mRNA (Samid *et al.*, 1985a). A gradual increase in the c-*ras*^{H} mRNA took place in the revertants following the cessation of IFN treatment (Samid *et al.*, 1985b). However, only a small fraction of these cells regained the transformed phenotype, while the majority remained non-transformed despite high levels of c-*ras*^{H} mRNA (persistent revertants). They transformed readily, however, following their treatment with 5-azacytidine (Friedman and Samid, personal communication). This agent causes DNA demethylation that in certain cases modulates the expression of cellular genes (reviewed by Hoffman, 1984). Since the c-*ras*^{H} was already expressed in these cells before the treatment, it is likely that the expression of genes other than the c-*ras*^{H} was affected by demethylation. These could be cellular genes involved in suppression of the transformed phenotype (Samid *et al.*, 1985b). The existence of such suppressor genes (anti-oncogenes) could also account for an additional interesting finding that the persistent revertants were also resistant to transformation with retroviruses carrying the v-*ras*^{K}, v-*ras*^{H}, v-*fos* and v-*abl* (Samid *et al.*, 1985a, c). Conversely, IFN could also repress cellular genes that render NIH 3T3 cells so highly susceptible to transformation (cooperating oncogenes?). These genes would remain silent even in the absence of IFN, but following their activation by 5-azacytidine could again cooperate with the c-*ras*^{H} in the transformation process.

The authors also studied the synthesis of the p21 protein in the original, revertant, and persistent revertant cells. In the revertant lines they found, by immunoprecipitation, a 4-fold reduction in the amount of p21 when compared to the original transformed cells, and suggested that the reduced level of p21 in the IFN-induced revertant cells might be involved in the IFN-induced phenotypic reversion from the transformed to the non-transformed state. Interestingly, the persistent revertants produced relatively high levels of p21, similar to the original transformed cells. Samid *et al.* (1985b, c) concluded that over-production of p21 in the persistent revertant cells alone is not sufficient to cause re-transformation.

In addition to the reversion of the transformed phenotype established by over-production of c-*ras*^{H}, IFN also inhibited the initiation of transformation with the EJ/T24 *ras*^{H} oncogene. This oncogene was isolated from a human bladder carcinoma and shown to be activated by a point mutation in the amino acid 12 of the *ras* p21 (Capon *et al.*, 1983). IFN treatment of mouse 3T3 cells transfected with this oncogene (and also with v-*ras*^{H} and v-*mos*) inhibited the development of transformed foci, even when applied 5–7 days after transfection (Samid *et al.*, 1985b). In this system the inhibition was specific only for the oncogenic transformation, as biochemical transformation with markers such as pSV2-neo or Ecogpt was not reduced. This is in contrast to the previously reported observations showing a general reduction of the transformation process by IFN (Otsuka *et al.*, 1982; Dubois *et al.*, 1983). Surprisingly, once the EJ/T24 *ras*^{H} transformation was established, IFN treatment was ineffective in reversing it. The authors speculated that this dichotomy could be explained by different threshold levels of p21 needed for transformation. Lower levels of the mutated p21 are needed for the induction of transformed phenotype as compared to the normal p21 (Feramisco *et al.*, 1984; Stacy and Kung, 1984). IFN-induced reduction in the level of p21 protein could therefore affect more profoundly the transformation established by the normal rather than the mutated c-*ras*^{H} oncogene.

D N-*ras*

The N-*ras* is one of the cellular oncogenes that does not have a direct counterpart among the known RNA tumour virus oncogenes. However, it is structurally and functionally related to the *ras* family of cellular and viral oncogenes. The N-*ras* has been identified by the NIH 3T3 assay as the transforming gene in DNAs from a variety of human tumours: carcinomas, sarcomas, neuroblastomas and in haematopoietic tumours (Shimizu *et al.*, 1983; Taparowsky *et al.*, 1983). The activation of transforming activity of N-*ras* has also been shown to be due to an amino acid substitution in the p21 N-*ras* protein (Yuasa *et al.*, 1984).

In Burkitt lymphoma DNA, it is the N-*ras* oncogene and not the c-*myc* that is responsible for the NIH 3T3 transformation (Murray *et al.*, 1983). As with the c-*myc* (see above), the N-*ras* expression has been shown to be regulated by IFN-β in the Burkitt lymphoma cell line Daudi, where it correlated and preceded the cessation of cell growth (Jonak *et al.*, 1985b). The N-*ras* and c-*myc* regulation, however, differed in two aspects. First, while the c-*myc* mRNA levels were regulated only quantitatively in both total and polysomal RNA, the N-*ras* mRNA was regulated quantitatively and qualitatively. In total RNA its electrophoretic mobility was decreased, while in the polysomal fraction both electrophoretic mobility and amount were reduced. The decrease in electrophoretic mobility suggests an increase in size that could be due to altered transcription and/or processing of the N-*ras* mRNA in IFN-treated cells. A decrease in the amount of the N-*ras* mRNA in the polysomal fraction indicates that it is also regulated in these cells at the translational level. Second, cycloheximide or emetine treatment abrogated the regulation of the N-*ras* but not of the c-*myc* mRNA. This suggests that new or sustained cellular protein synthesis is needed for the regulation of the N-*ras* but not the c-*myc* gene.

E Other oncogenes

In addition to the above oncogenes, whose regulation by IFN has been analysed in more detail, it is also worthwhile to present preliminary data from other systems for which the analyses are underway. An IFN-dependent reduction in cellular RNA hybridizable to a v-*src* probe (the oncogene of

Raus sarcoma virus) has been reported by Soslau *et al.* (1984). The cells used in this study were the growth-arrested human bladder carcinoma cells (RT4) employed for the analysis of the c-*ras*^{H} oncogene (see above). The authors have also noted in these IFN-treated cells a reduction in quantity and modification of a phosphorylatable protein (p60) that, at least in size, was analogous to the p60 v-*src* protein. It remains to be determined whether this cellular p60 protein is antigenically related to the viral *src* p60.

An IFN-mediated down-regulation of the p53 cellular oncogene was recently reported (Kimchi *et al.*, 1985a). This oncogene has no known viral counterpart and codes for a metabolically labile protein of 53,000 daltons that may play a role in cell proliferation. This notion is based on findings that the p53 mRNA and protein were induced in fibroblasts and lymphocytes stimulated to proliferate with growth factors (Reich *et al.*, 1983). In addition, microinjection of anti-p53 antibody abrogated the induction of DNA synthesis in serum-stimulated quiescent fibroblasts (Mercer *et al.*, 1983). The p53 expression leads to immortalization of primary cells *in vitro* and renders them sensitive to transformation with *ras* oncogenes (Parada *et al.*, 1984). The level of p53 protein was reduced by 70% in Daudi cells treated with 100 units/ml of human IFN-α. The reduction correlated with the growth state of the cells, since it was evident only in a line of Daudi cells whose growth was inhibited by IFN-α, but not in the Daudi line that was resistant to the anti-proliferative action of IFN-α (Kimchi *et al.*, 1985a).

A reduction in the steady-state level of cellular mRNA complementary to the Moloney sarcoma virus oncogene (v-*mos*) was detected in Daudi cells treated with anti-proliferative but not anti-viral doses of IFN (Krueger *et al.*, 1984). The anti-viral dose of IFN rendered the cells "super-sensitive", however, and the additional dose of even 1 unit/ml of IFN caused a rapid cessation of cell growth and the c-*mos* mRNA reduction. The authors speculated that different doses of IFN regulate the expression of different banks of cellular genes. The gene bank, including the c-*mos* and possibly other c-*onc*, would be regulated and play a role only in the anti-proliferative but not the anti-viral response induced by IFN (Krueger *et al.*, 1984; Carter *et al.*, 1985). Of interest is a preliminary clinical report that the expression of c-*abl* oncogene (cellular homologue of Abelson murine sarcoma virus oncogene, v-*abl*) was reduced in blood cells of two chronic leukemia patients treated with high doses of natural human IFN-α (Carter *et al.*, 1985).

IV FUTURE CHALLENGES AND PROSPECTS

> False facts are highly injurious to the progress of science, for they often endure long; but false views, if supported by some evidence, do little harm, for everyone takes a salutary pleasure in proving their falseness. *Charles Darwin*

The investigation of the expression of c-*onc* in response to IFNs should increase our understanding of their regulation and function at both the cellular and molecular levels. As summarized in this review, the available experimental data clearly demonstrate that IFNs have the capacity to repress certain c-*onc* not only in normal cells but also in tumour cells. In several experimental systems, the c-*onc* repression correlates with the IFN-mediated cessation of cell growth or with the inhibition of establishment or maintenance of transformed phenotype. The modulation of c-*onc* expression appears therefore to be related to some of the anti-cellular effects of IFN. However, the available experimental data are at present fragmentary and even conflicting, thus not yet permitting more definite assessment of the crucial question whether the c-*onc* modulation is the cause of, consequence of, or an event completely unrelated to, the anti-cellular effects of IFN. What type of experimental strategies might therefore yield more definite answers and reconcile some of the conflicting reports on the presence or absence of c-*onc* modulation by IFNs?

Undoubtedly, studies in the areas of cell and cancer biology dealing with the role of oncogenes in cell growth regulation, differentiation and the process of neoplastic transformation are parallel research endeavours, and IFN research will benefit from these experiments. The studies with mutant cells whose growth regulation and c-*onc* expression *vis-à-vis* IFN are different from the parental cells (Einat *et al.*, 1985b; Knight *et al.*, 1985b; Dron *et al.*, 1985), and with somatic cell hybrids between IFN-sensitive and resistant cells (Kimchi *et al.*, 1985b, c), have the potential for further defining the roles of c-*onc* at the cellular level and should be pursued. While most of the studies thus far have dealt with the anti-cellular effect of exogenously added IFN, it has also been suggested the endogenously produced IFN, and cellular functions regulated by it (such as c-*onc*), may play a role in certain terminal differentiation events (Resnitsky *et al.*, 1985) and serve as a feedback regulator for the action of growth factors (Zullo *et al.*, 1985). Results derived from such systems should also be very informative.

The list of oncogenes continues to grow and it is being recognized that more than one oncogene may be required for events regulating growth and functions of normal and tumour cells (Kelly *et al.*, 1983; Land *et al.*, 1983). The oncogenic products may interact with each other or with other cellular genes in a cascade-like manner or function in converging parallel pathways in order to regulate or execute cellular processes. The elements of these interactions may vary from cell type to cell type, and also the sensitivity of the different elements to IFN-mediated regulation may not be the same among cells. It would be an expression of terminal naiveté to assume that one oncogene or one mechanism will account for the anti-cellular activity of various IFNs. After all, it is generally accepted that no single mechanism and locus of action can account for or play a predominant role in the anti-viral mechanisms induced by IFN. Therefore, it may be necessary at times to use a rather brutal approach and investigate in a single cell type the effect of IFN on the expression of more than one known oncogene and/or to include in the investigation newly-discovered oncogenes.

The current and most straightforward approach to studying IFN's role in the expression of oncogenes has been to compare the steady-state levels of mRNA and/or proteins of an oncogene in control and IFN-treated cells. The molecular mechanisms of IFN-induced regulation may be multiple and more subtle than gross changes in the levels of mRNA or proteins. An altered compartmentalization or translatability of mRNA would result in a decreased level of an oncogenic protein, but would not be detected at the level of total mRNA. Minor changes in processing, modification or subcellular localization of an oncogenic product in IFN-treated cells may not be readily detectable with current methodology, yet they may all profoundly affect the functional properties of c-*onc* proteins. Multiple experimental approaches will have to be made that utilize more sophisticated measurements than are used at present.

A considerable part of the experimental efforts in this area will certainly be devoted to the mechanism(s) of c-*onc* regulation—specifically, how they relate to the cellular functions known to be induced by IFN—and for the purpose of discovering new regulatory factors. The involvement of the 2–5A synthetase-RNase L system activated by double-stranded regions of the c-*myc* mRNA has been suggested as one mechanism that may play a role in its post-transcriptional regulation (Knight *et al.*, 1985a). Comparisons of the stability and translatability of mRNAs from structurally altered c-*onc* transfected into IFN-sensitive cells should aid in determining whether certain structural features in mRNAs play a role in their regulation by IFN. Even a more advanced approach, used successfully for other cellular genes, will involve the development of systems entirely *in vitro*, capable of analysing and dissecting the IFN mechanism. This would make the identification and isolation of specific effector molecules more feasible and amenable to detailed analysis at the molecular level. In fact, an *in vitro* system is being developed for analysing the mechanisms of the transcriptional regulation of c-*myc* by IFN (Yarden and Kimchi, 1985). The rationale here is to identify nuclear proteins that bind to the c-*myc* upstream sequences and negatively regulate its transcription. The mechanism of the c-ras^{H} regulation (Samid *et al.*, 1985a) could also be analysed with this method.

As reviewed recently by Gresser (1985), correlations between the effects of IFN on tumour cell growth in culture and the effects of IFN on the growth of the same tumour cells in an animal are not always obvious. Therefore, as Gresser suggested, the mechanism of cell growth inhibition by IFN on cells in culture may be different from that on the same cells in an animal. Hence, in addition to the study of IFN-mediated c-*onc* regulation in tissue culture cells, equally important will be the recently initiated research on the IFN-induced modulation of c-*onc* in animal tumours and cancer patients (Samid *et al.*, 1985b, c; Glasgow *et al.*, 1985; Carter *et al.*, 1985). This type of research will be considerably more difficult, since it will have to deal not only with the regulation of c-*onc* involved in the unregulated growth of tumour cells, but also with the immense complexity of entire organisms, including the immune response, and with the metastatic properties of cancer cells. The recent discovery of cellular genes conferring metastatic potential (Bernstein and Weinberg, 1985) should aid in this endeavour.

If a role for c-*onc* in the regulation of cell functions is established, it is likely to be complex. At present, generalizations are dangerous and may not be possible. Simple solutions are not the norm for complex organisms and that is a benefit for those of us doing research. A single experiment or group of experiments will be unlikely to provide a unified and satisfactory explanation for IFN action. Complexity in cellular regulation exists in the prokaryotes, so we will have to be ready to deal with much more complexity in growth regulation in the higher organisms. "My mechanism is *the* mechanism" will probably no longer be useful. Multiple regulatory sites are everywhere, and it is informative to remember that not much more than a decade ago we thought there was only one human IFN.

ACKNOWLEDGEMENTS

We thank our colleagues Elizabeth D. Anton, Diana Fahey, and Barbara K. Friedland for collaboration in our research on IFN and oncogenes. We appreciate the manuscript and abstracts sent to us by R. Friedman, D. Gillespie, J. Kelly, A. Kimchi, B. Lebleu, P. Lengyel, and D. Samid. We thank Bruce D. Korant for a critical reading of this review, and Betty B. Wolfe for typing and assembling the manuscript.

REFERENCES

Armelin, H. A., Armelin, M. C. S., Kelly, K., Stewart, T., Leder, P., Cochran, B. H. and Stiles, C. D. (1984). *Nature (London)* **310**, 655–660.

Bernstein, S. C. and Weinberg, R. A. (1985). *Proc. Natl Acad. Sci. USA* **82**, 1726–1730.

Bishop, J. M. (1981). *Cell* **23**, 5–6.

Bishop, J. M. (1983) *Ann. Rev. Biochem.* **52**, 301–354.

Blair, D. G., Cooper, C. S., Oskarsson, M. K., Eader, L. A. and Vande Woude, G. F. (1982). *Science* **218**, 1122–1125.

Capon, D. J., Seeburg, P. H., McGrath, J. P., Hayflick, J. S., Edman, U., Levinson, A. D., and Goeddel, D. V. (1983). *Nature* (*London*) **304**, 507–512.
Carter, W. A., Swartz, H. and Gillespie, D. H. (1985). *J. Biol. Response Modif.* (in press).
Chang, E. H., Furth, M. E., Scolnick, E. M. and Lowy, D. R. (1982). *Nature* (*London*) **297**, 479–483.
Chany, C. and Vignal, M. (1970). *J. Gen. Virol.* **7**, 203–210.
Clemens, M. J. and McNurlan, M. A. (1985). *Biochem. J.* **226**, 345–360.
Collins, S. and Groudine, M. (1982). *Nature* (*London*) **298**, 679–681.
Cooper, G. M. and Lane, M.-A. (1984). *Biochim. Biophys. Acta* **738**, 9–20.
Cooper, G. M., Okenquist, S. and Silverman, L. (1980). *Nature* (*London*) **284**, 418–421.
Corcoran, L. M., Adams, J. M., Dunn, A. R. and Cory, S. (1984). *Cell* **37**, 113–122.
Curran, T., Peters, G., Van Beveren, C., Teich, N. M. and Verma, I. M. (1982). *J. Virol.* **44**, 674–682.
Dani, C., Mechti, N., Piechaczyk, M., Lebleu, B., Jeanteur, P. and Blanchard, J. M. (1985). *Proc. Natl Acad. Sci. USA* **82**, 4896–4899.
DeFeo-Jones, D., Scolnick, E. M., Koller, R. and Dhar, R. (1983). *Nature* (*London*) **306**, 707–709
Dony, C., Kessel, M. and Gruss, P. (1985). *Nature* (*London*) **317**, 636–639.
Downward, J., Yarden, Y., Mayes, E., Scrace, G., Totty, N., Stockwell, P., Ullrich, A., Schlessinger, J. and Waterfield, M. D. (1984). *Nature* (*London*) **307**, 521–527.
Dron, M. and Tovey, M. G. (1983) *J. Gen. Virol.* **64**, 2641–2647.
Dron, M., Modjtahedi, Brison, O. and Tovey, M. G. (1986) *Molec. Cell Biol.* **6**, 1374–1378.
Dubois, M. F., Vignal, M., LeCunff, M. and Chany, C. (1983). *Nature* (*London*) **303**, 433–435.
Duesberg, P. H. (1983). *Nature* (*London*) **304**, 219–226.
Duesberg, P. H. (1985). *Science* **228**, 669–677.
Einat, M., Resnitzky, D. and Kimchi, A. (1985a). *Proc. Natl Acad. Sci. USA* **82**, 7608–7612.
Einat, M., Resnitzky, D. and Kimchi, A. (1985b). *Nature* (*London*) **313**, 597–600.
Feramisco, J. R., Gross, M., Kamata, T., Rosenberg, M. and Sweet, R. W. (1984). *Cell* **38**, 109–117.
Gibbs, J. B., Sigal, I. S., Poe, M. and Scolnick, E. M. (1984). *Proc. Natl Acad. Sci. USA* **81**, 5704–5708.
Glasgow, G., Wivel, N. A. and Pitha, P. M. (1985). Abstract, p. 102, TNO-ISIR Meeting on the Interferon System, Clearwater Beach, Florida, USA.
Greenberg, M. E. and Ziff, E. B. (1984). *Nature* (*London*) **311**, 433–438.
Gresser, I. (ed.). (1985). *In* "Interferon 6", pp. 93–126. Academic Press, New York.
Hann, S. R. and Eisenman, R. N. (1984). *Molec. Cell. Biol.* **4**, 2486–2497.
Hann, S. R., Thompson, C. B. and Eisenman, R. N. (1985). *Nature* (*London*) **314**, 366–369.
Hayward, W. C., Neel, B. G. and Astrin, S. M. (1981). *Nature* (*London*) **290**, 475–480.
Hoffman, R. M. (1984). *Biochim. Biophys. Acta* **738**, 49–87.
Inglot, A. D., Oleszak, E. and Kisielow, B. (1980). *Arch. Virol.* **63**, 291–296.
Jonak, G. J. and Knight, E., Jr. (1984). *Proc. Natl Acad. Sci. USA* **81**, 1747–1750.
Jonak, G. J., Anton, E. D., Fahey, D., Friedland, B. K., Cheng, Y.-S. and Knight, E. Jr. (1985a). *In* "The Biology of the Interferon System 1984" H. Kirchner and H. Schellekens, eds.), pp. 205–212. Elsevier, Amsterdam.

Jonak, G. J., Friedland, B. K., Anton, E. D., Fahey, D. and Knight, E. Jr. (1985b). Abstract, p. 31, TNO-ISIR Meeting on the Interferon System, Clearwater Beach, Florida, USA.

Kaczmarek, L., Hyland, J. K., Watt, R., Rosenberg, M. and Baserga, R. (1985). *Science* **228**, 1313–1315.

Kelly, J. M., Gilbert, C. S., Stark, G. S. and Kerr, I. M. (1985). *Eur. J. Biochem.* **153**, 367–371.

Kelly, K. and Siebenlist, U. (1985). *J. Clin. Immunol.* **5**, 65–77.

Kelly, K., Cochran, B. H., Stiles, C. D. and Leder, P. (1983). *Cell* **35**, 603–610.

Kimchi, A., Resnitzky, D., Bendori, R. and Einat, M. (1985a). *In* "The Biology of the Interferon System 1984" (H. Kirchner and H. Schellekens, eds.), pp. 205–212. Elsevier, Amsterdam.

Kimchi, A., Yarden, A., Gat, G. and Resnitzky, D. (1985b). *In* "Proceedings of the Sixth International Symposium of the Research Institute: The 2-5A System" (B. R. G. Williams and R. H. Silverman, eds.). Allan Liss, Inc., New York (in press).

Kimchi, A., Resnitzky, D., Einat, M., Yarden, A. and Gat, G. (1985c). Abstract, p. 29, TNO-ISIR Meeting on the Interferon System, Clearwater Beach, Florida, USA.

Knight, E., Jr., Anton, E. D., Fahey, D., Friedland, B. K. and Jonak, G. (1985a). *Proc. Natl Acad. Sci. USA* **82**, 1151–1154.

Knight, E., Jr., Friedland, B. K., Anton, E. D., Fahey, D. and Jonak, G. J. (1985b.) *In* "The Interferon System" (F. Dianzani and G. D. Rossi, eds.), pp. 405–413. Raven Press, New York.

Krueger, L. J., Bresser, J., Andryuk, P. J. and Gillespie, D. H. (1984). *J. Cell. Biochem. Supp.* **8A**, 85.

Land, H., Parada, L. F. and Weinberg, R. A. (1983). *Nature* (*London*) **304**, 596–602.

McGrath, J. P., Capon, D. J., Goeddel, D. V. and Levinson, A. D. (1984). *Nature* (*London*) **310**, 644–649.

Mercer, W. E., Nelson, D., DeLeo, A. B., Old, L. J. and Baserga, R. (1982). *Proc. Natl Acad. Sci. USA* **79**, 6309–6312.

Miller, A. D., Curan, T. and Verma, I. M. (1984). *Cell* **36**, 51–60.

Müller, R., Müller, A. D., and Guilbert, L. (1984a) *EMBO J.* **3**, 1887–1890.

Müller, R., Bravo, R., Burckhardt, J. and Curran, T. (1984b). *Nature* (*London*) **312**, 716–720.

Müller, R. and Wagner, E. F. (1984) *Nature* (*London*) **311**, 438–442.

Murray, M. J., Cunningham, J. M., Parada, L. F., Dautry, F., Lebowitz, P. and Weinberg, R. A. (1983) *Cell* **33**, 749–757.

Otsuka, H., Qavi, H. and Kit, S. (1982). *Antiviral Res.* **2**, 301–311.

Parada, L. F., Land, H., Weinberg, R. A., Wolf, D. and Rotter, V. (1984). *Nature* (*London*) **312**, 649–651.

Paucker, K., Cantell, K. and Henle, W. (1962). *Virology* **17**, 324–338.

Persson, H. and Leder, P. (1984). *Science* **225**, 718–721.

Persson, H., Hennighausen, L., Taub, R., DeGrado, W. and Leder, P. (1984). *Science* **225**, 687–693.

Ramsay, G., Evan, G. I. and Bishop (1984). *Proc. Natl Acad. Sci. USA* **81**, 7742–7746.

Reich, N. C., Oren, M. and Levine, A. J. (1983). *Molec. Cell Biol.* **3**, 2143–2150.

Reitsma, P. H., Rothberg, P. G., Astrin, S. M., Trial, J., Bar-Shavit, Z., Hall, A., Teitelbaum, S. L. and Kahn, A. J. (1983). *Nature* (*London*) **306**, 492–494.

Resnitzky, D., Zipori, D. and Kimchi, A. (1985). Abstract, p. 117, TNO-ISIR Meeting on the Interferon System, Clearwater Beach, Florida, USA.

Salehzada, T., Blanchard, J. M., Mechti, N., Piechaczyk, M., Dani, C., Jeanteur, P. and Lebleu, B. (1985). *In* "Proceedings of the Sixth International Symposium of the Research Institute: The 2-5A System" (B. R. G. Williams and R. H. Silverman, eds.). Alan Liss, Inc., New York (in press).

Samid, D., Chang, E. H. and Friedman, R. M. (1984). *Biochem. Biophys. Res. Commun.* **119**, 21–28.

Samid, D., Chang, E. H. and Friedman, R. M. (1985a). Abstract, RNA Tumor Virus Meeting, Cold Spring Harbor Laboratory.

Samid, D., Flessate, D. M., Greene, J. J., Chang, E. H. and Friedman, R. M. (1985b). *In* "Proceedings of the Sixth International Symposium of the Research Institute: The 2-5A System" (B. R. G. Williams and R. H. Silverman, eds.). Alan Liss, Inc., New York, (in press).

Samid, D., Chang, E. H. and Friedman, R. M. (1985c). Abstract, p. 19, TNO-ISIR Meeting on the Interferon System, Clearwater Beach, Florida, USA.

Shen-Ong, G. L. C., Keath, E. J., Piccoli, S. P. and Cole, M. D. (1982). *Cell* **31**, 443–452.

Shih, C., Shilo, B.-Z., Goldfarb, M. P., Dannenberg, A. and Weinberg, R. A. (1979). *Proc. Natl Acad. Sci. USA* **76**, 5714–5718.

Shilo, B.-Z. and Weinberg, R. A. (1981). *Proc. Natl Acad. Sci. USA* **78**, 6789–6792.

Shimizu, K., Goldfarb, M., Suard, Y., Peruclio, M., Li, Y., Kamata, T., Feramisco, J., Stavnezer, E., Fogh, J. and Wigler, M. H. (1983). *Proc. Natl Acad. Sci. USA* **80**, 2112–2116.

Soslau, G., Bogucki, A. R., Gillespie, D. and Hubbel, H. R. (1984). *Biochem. Biophys. Res. Commun.* **119**, 941–948.

Stacey, D. W. and Kung, H. F. (1984). *Nature* (*London*) **310**, 508–511.

Taparowsky, E., Shimizu, K., Goldfarb, M. and Wigler, M. (1983). *Cell* **34**, 581–586.

Taub, R., Kirsch, I., Morton, C., Lenoir, G., Swan, D., Tronick, S., Aaronson, S. and Leder, P. (1982). *Proc. Natl Acad. Sci. USA* **79**, 7837–7841.

Thompson, C. B., Challoner, P. B., Neiman, P. E. and Groudine, M. (1985). *Nature* (*London*) **314**, 363–366.

Todaro, G. J. and Green, H. (1967). *J. Virol.* **1**, 115–119.

Tominaga, S. and Lengyel, P. (1985). *J. Biol. Chem.* **260**, 1975–1978.

Verma, I. M., Curran, T., Müller, R., van Straaten, F., MacConnell, W., Miller, A. D. and Van Beveren, C. (1984). *In* "Cancer Cell 2" (G. Vande Woude, A. J. Levine, W. C. Topp and J. D. Watson, eds.), pp. 309–321. Cold Spring Harbor, New York.

Waterfield, M. D., Scrace, G. T., Whittle, N., Stroobant, P., Johnsson, A., Wasteson, A., Westermark, B., Heldin, C.-H., Huang, J. S. and Deuel, T. F. (1983). *Nature* (*London*) **304**, 35–39.

Weinberg, R. A. (1985). *Science* **230**, 770–776.

Yarden, A. and Kimchi, A. (1985). Abstract, p. 84, TNO-ISIR Meeting on the Interferon System, Clearwater Beach, Florida, USA.

Yuasa, Y., Gol, R. A., Chang, A., Chiu, I.-M., Reddy, E. P., Tronick, S. R. and Aaronson, S. A. (1984). *Proc. Natl Acad. Sci. USA* **81**, 3670–3674.

Zullo, J., Cochran, B. H., Huang, A. S. and Stiles, C. D. (1985). Abstract, p. 237, First Annual Meeting on Oncogenes, Hood College, Frederick, MD, USA.

AIDS and Kaposi's Sarcoma: Interferons in Pathogenesis and Treatment

SUSAN E. KROWN

Clinical Immunology Service, Department of Medicine, Memorial Sloan-Kettering Cancer Center, New York, NY 10021, USA

It is probably not hyperbolic to begin this essay by saying that never has a disease so captured the interest, concern and imagination of the scientific community and lay public as has the acquired immunodeficiency syndrome (AIDS). First described in 1981 (Centers for Disease Control, 1981 a, b; Gottlieb *et al.*, 1981; Masur *et al.*, 1981; Siegal *et al.*, 1981) in a small number of young male homosexuals and users of intravenous narcotics, AIDS has now, in the fall of 1985, been reported in over 14,000 people in the United States and in countries around the globe. Among those affected have been elderly transfusion recipients, haemophiliacs, women and children, in addition to the two groups originally identified which, between them, account for close to 90% of the reported cases. Current estimates of the number of people who have been infected with the presumed aetiological virus, HTLV-III/LAV

INTERFERON 7
ISBN 0 12 302256 8

(Barré-Sinoussi *et al.*, 1983; Gallo *et al.*, 1984), range from the hundreds of thousands to over a million (Sivak and Wormser, 1985), but it is by no means clear what proportion of such individuals will eventually develop the full-blown syndrome.

The medical spectrum of AIDS-associated illnesses is such that physicians from almost every medical specialty and subspecialty have become involved in the treatment of AIDS patients. Similarly, scientists from a wide range of disciplines—virologists, immunologists, molecular biologists, epidemiologists, to name a few—have contributed to our understanding of the aetiology, transmission and physiopathology of the disease. The devastating consequences of the disease, coupled with confusion and misinformation about its mode of spread and its contagiousness, have led to fear and often hysteria among parents, teachers, school boards and sexually active heterosexuals. The intense emotional and social pressures attendant upon the disease have required the involvement of psychiatrists, social workers and the clergy, and the financial burdens of catastrophic illness in often young and unprepared individuals have placed enormous burdens on patients and their families as well as government and private agencies. In one way or another, AIDS has affected essentially every stratum and corner of society, and it is not an unusual day on which I rise to hear a radio news item about AIDS, care for patients with AIDS in the afternoon, see a headline about AIDS in the evening paper, and retire after an 11 o'clock TV news report about AIDS.

My entrée into the many-faceted world of AIDS was via interferon, and it is to that subject—the relationship of AIDS to the interferon system and the role of interferon in the treatment of some of its manifestations—that I devote the remainder of this chapter. Although my initial approach to the disease was from the relatively narrow perspective of an oncologist intent upon evaluating the activity of interferon alpha against a tumour occurring in patients with an unnamed and only partially characterized constellation of signs and symptoms, it has since become clear that the interferon system, and in particular perturbations in that system, may play an important role in our understanding of the physiopathology of AIDS and suggest new approaches to its treatment.

I BACKGROUND

A The Acquired Immunodeficiency Syndrome (AIDS)

Although it is beyond the scope of this essay to describe in detail the many manifestations of AIDS, it is important to define the scope of the syndrome and to mention those manifestations that relate to later discussion of interferons. For surveillance purposes, the Centers for Disease Control (CDC) originally defined AIDS as the presence of a reliably diagnosed disease at least moderately indicative of underlying cellular immunodeficiency occurring in the absence of known causes of underlying immunodeficiency or host defence defect (e.g. immunosuppressive therapy or pre-existing lymphoreticular malignancy) (Centers for Disease Control, 1982). The diseases encompassed by this definition included Kaposi's sarcoma in patients less than 60 years of age, primary lymphomas of the central nervous system and a variety of so-called "opportunistic infections" that do not occur in exposed but immunocompetent individuals. Common among the many such infections are *Pneumocystis carinii* pneumonia, disseminated infection with *Mycobacterim avium-intracellulare* and central nervous system infection with *Toxoplasma gondii.* These three infections are of particular interest in the context of a discussion of interferons because of the role of macrophages in host defence against them, a feature which will be discussed later.

AIDS was operationally defined for reporting purposes before its aetiology was known, and the definition therefore encompassed only certain secondary conditions that reliably reflected the presence of a severe immune dysfunction. More recently, with the recognition of HTLV-III/LAV as the cause of AIDS and the development of laboratory tests to detect antibody to the aetiological virus, it has become possible to include additional conditions in the definition of the syndrome and to improve the specificity of the definition used for reporting cases (Centers for Disease Control, 1985).

Patients with "full-blown" AIDS and those classified as having the so-called "AIDS-related complex" differ in that the latter group, while having many of the signs and symptoms associated with AIDS, do not manifest the typical opportunistic infections or tumours that define the full-blown syndrome. Although such patients have an increased incidence of developing AIDS, it is not clear what proportion of such patients will eventually develop the syndrome. Many, but not all, of these signs and symptoms—generalized lymphadenopathy, unintentional weight loss, fever, chronic diarrhoea, malaise, lethargy, lymphopenia, leukopenia, anemia, idiopathic thrombocytopenia, immunological abnormalities and oral candidiasis—are similar to those reported after administration of exogenous interferons to patients with other diseases, a point which will be emphasized later.

B Kaposi's Sarcoma

More than a century ago Moritz Kaposi, a Hungarian dermatologist practising in Vienna, published the first description of the "multiple idiopathic pigmented sarcomas of the skin" that now bear his name (Kaposi, 1872). He described five men between the ages of 50 and 70 who had multiple vascular nodules in the skin, and noted that the disease could appear simultaneously in more than one part of the body and could, on occasion, involve visceral organs.

Until its recognition as the tumour most frequently associated with AIDS, Kaposi's sarcoma was relatively rare in the western world, with an estimated annual incidence in the United States of 0.02 to 0.06 per 100,000 (Oettle, 1962; Reynolds *et al.*, 1965). Despite its rarity, certain unique features of this tumour have long made Kaposi's sarcoma a subject of interest to investigators from a wide range of disciplines, including epidemiology, genetics, virology and immunology. Such investigations provided a rationale for the use of interferon in AIDS-associated Kaposi's sarcoma, and for study of the interferon system in AIDS patients, long before full characterization of the disease and discovery of the aetiological virus.

Prior to its association with AIDS, Kaposi's sarcoma was diagnosed most often among Central and Eastern Europeans, Italians, and blacks from Equatorial Africa (see Safai and Good, 1980). In North America, most patients have been, by birth or descent, Italians or Jews from Eastern Europe and Russia. Such geographical and ethnic clustering of cases suggests a role for genetic or environmental factors; familial cases have, however, been observed only rarely (Oettle, 1962; Lothe, 1963; Epstein, 1972). Although patients from diverse ethnic and racial backgrounds have developed Kaposi's sarcoma in association with AIDS, patients with both the "classical" and "epidemic" forms of the disease have been shown to have an increased frequency of the HLA-DR5 antigen, suggesting that common genetic factors may be involved in susceptibility to this tumour (Friedman-Kien *et al.*, 1982; Pollack *et al.*, 1983; Metroka *et al.*, 1983). The importance of genetic susceptibility, as opposed to environmental and geographic factors, is also suggested by the observation that among certain South African Bantus the incidence of Kaposi's sarcoma is 10 times that observed in the white population of the same area (Keen, 1962). (This argument is weakened, however, when one considers that the living environment of the Bantus may differ significantly from that of white South Africans. A situation comparable to that observed for polio virus infection can be envisioned, with individuals living in crowded, poor sanitation areas generally being exposed in early childhood to the aetiological agent, and those living in areas with good sanitation and better living standards being exposed less frequently and at a later age. In the case of paralytic poliomyelitis, good living conditions may be a disadvantage; if one hypothesizes an aetiological "agent" for Kaposi's sarcoma, the reverse may apply.)

The high incidence of Kaposi's sarcoma in certain geographical areas, particularly in Africa, has indeed suggested a role for an infectious agent in the pathogenesis of the disease. Parallels have been drawn between the geographical clustering of Kaposi's sarcoma and that of Burkitt's lymphoma in Africa, where a strong association with a transforming herpes virus, the Epstein-Barr virus, has been clearly established. However, the geographical distribution of these two neoplasms is not identical. Giraldo *et al.* (1972) reported herpes-type virus particles in cell lines derived from African patients with Kaposi's sarcoma. Subsequent investigations by Giraldo and coworkers demonstrated an apparent association between Kaposi's sarcoma and antibodies to cytomegalovirus (CMV) in Africans and Europeans (Giraldo *et al.*, 1975) and in North American patients (Giraldo *et al.*, 1978). Although these data suggest a link between CMV infection and the development of Kaposi's sarcoma, an aetiological role for the virus has not been established.

It has been hypothesized, however, that persistent infection with CMV in genetically susceptible and immunobiologically responsive individuals may lead to neoplastic transformation and the development of Kaposi's sarcoma (Safai *et al.*, 1980). The almost universal detection of high-titre antibodies to CMV in patients with AIDS-associated Kaposi's sarcoma and the frequent isolation of CMV from the blood and secretions of such patients (Gelmann *et al.*, 1985) supports the concept of persistent CMV infection in such individuals, but by no means establishes an aetiological role for the virus. Perhaps more compelling evidence in support of a role for CMV is the observation that heterosexual patients with AIDS, who develop Kaposi's sarcoma far less frequently than homosexual men with the syndrome, have an incidence of antibodies to CMV that more closely approximates that of the normal adult population (J. W. M. Gold, personal communication). The available evidence does not support a direct role for HTLV-III/LAV in the aetiology of AIDS-related Kaposi's sarcoma, as viral DNA sequences have not been detected in any Kaposi's sarcoma tumour specimens, but have been found in many other tissues from such patients (Shaw *et al.*, 1984; Hahn, 1985).

The role of the immune system in the development and clinical course of Kaposi's sarcoma also received considerable attention prior to the recognition of AIDS. The increased frequency of Kaposi's sarcoma in individuals receiving immunosuppressive drugs (Harwood *et al.*, 1979; Klein *et al.*, 1974; Myers *et al.*, 1974), and the well-documented "spontaneous" regression of Kaposi's sarcoma in kidney transplant patients in whom immunosuppressive therapy was withdrawn, imply a role for immunological mechanisms in the genesis of the tumour and suggest that an intact immune system can, of itself, lead to tumour control. In certain African patients with highly aggressive forms of Kaposi's sarcoma, cellular immune function was found to be severely impaired, whereas in those with more indolent forms of the disease, immune function was more nearly intact (Master *et al.*, 1970; Taylor, 1973;

Taylor and Ziegler, 1974). In this regard it is noteworthy that many patients with AIDS-associated Kaposi's sarcoma have a clinical picture that has been likened to the more aggressive African forms of the tumour, although the presentation of the disease differs in a number of respects (for a review, see Krown, 1984). Patients with classical European and North American Kaposi's sarcoma have shown an unusually high incidence of second primary malignancies, particularly those of the lymphoreticular system (Moertel, 1966; Oettle, 1963; Rothman, 1962; Safai *et al.*, 1980), suggesting that these tumours share related aetiopathogenic mechanisms. Similarly, in patients with AIDS, an increased incidence of various histological types of malignant lymphoma, including Burkitt's lymphoma (Ziegler *et al.*, 1982) immunoblastic lymphoma (Snider *et al.*, 1983), lymphoblastic lymphoma (Ciobanu, *et al.*, 1983) and Hodgkin's disease (Longo, 1984), has been observed.

The suggestive but indirect evidence supporting a role for a virus in the aetiology of Kaposi's sarcoma, the compelling evidence for immune dysfunction in its pathogenesis, and the recognition that Kaposi's sarcoma represents a neoplastic proliferation of cells, all provided a rationale for trials of an agent that possessed at once antiviral, immunomodulatory and antiproliferative properties. In 1981 the use of interferon against Kaposi's sarcoma seemed to embody the most rational approach to the disease. Its simplicity and logic seemed almost too good to be true. The plot thickened later, but fortunately not before we had already achieved some modest success. Had we understood then some of the features of AIDS that subsequently came to light, we might have hesitated to use interferon. Ignorance, as it turned out, while not quite blissful, permitted some interesting observations—but more about that later.

II THE INTERFERON SYSTEM IN AIDS

A Deficiencies of Interferon Production

Perhaps the most compelling argument in favour of interferons as potential therapeutic agents in AIDS comes from studies demonstrating deficiencies in the ability of cells from AIDS patients to produce normal amounts of both alpha and gamma interferons. Such deficiencies, it has been hypothesized, may explain the marked predisposition of such patients to opportunistic infections.

1 Interferon α

Lopez *et al.* (1983, 1984) reasoned that a defect in mononuclear cell generation of IFN-α might explain the increased susceptibility of AIDS patients to severe viral infections, particularly chronic ulcerative infections with *Herpes simplex* virus (HSV) (Siegal *et al.*, 1981). Whereas a subpopulation of mononuclear cells from normal individuals generates large quantities of acid-stable IFN-α when co-cultured with HSV-1 infected fibroblasts, many patients with AIDS or the AIDS-related complex showed a marked deficiency of IFN-α generation (Lopez *et al.*, 1983, 1984). Deficient IFN-α generation was, in turn, associated with an increased risk of developing opportunistic infection within a relatively brief follow-up period. That the deficiency of IFN-α-generating capacity may be causally related to susceptibility to infection, rather than a consequence of established infection, is suggested by the finding that patients without AIDS who were studied during acute viral or mycobacterial infections showed a normal capacity to produce IFN-α *in vitro*. Confirmatory evidence indicating a defect in IFN-α production has been obtained using different inducers by Gerstoft *et al.* (1982) and by Abb *et al.* (1984)

The findings of Lopez *et al.* have also been confirmed by Hersh *et al.* (1985), who cultured peripheral blood mononuclear cells with heat-inactivated preparations of HSV-1, HSV-2 and CMV and measured lymphocyte proliferative responses, NK cell activitation and IFN-α production in the cultures. Compared to normal controls, the cells from patients with AIDS and the AIDS-related complex showed significantly lower interferon induction (particularly in response to HSV-1 and -2), and a lesser degree of boosting of NK cell activity. The lymphocyte proliferative response was stimulated to a greater extent in normal controls' cells than in patients' cells only by HSV-1, but not by HSV-2 or CMV. Interestingly, the addition of interleukin-2 to the cultures consistently increased NK activity and blastogenic responses of patients' cells, but increased the interferon response only sporadically. Of potential relevance in this context is a preliminary report by Ikossi-O'Connor *et al.* (1984) indicating IFN-α-inactivating activity in the serum of some patients with AIDS. Although the nature of the inactivating activity has not been defined, it is noteworthy that the addition of antibody to IFN-α to IL-2-stimulated cells from patients with AIDS has been reported, in some cases, to reinitiate the release of HTLV-III in cultures no longer producing virus (Gallo *et al.*, 1984).

2 *Interferon γ*

The opportunistic pathogens regularly encountered in AIDS patients—protozoa (*P. carinii* and *T. gondii*), mycobacteria (*M. avium-intracellulare, M. tuberculosis*), viruses (HSV, CMV), fungi (*Candida albicans, Cryptococcus neoformans, Histoplasma capsulatum*), and, to a lesser extent, bacteria (*Listeria monocytogenes*, for example)—all require intact cell-mediated immune responses for effective control (Wing and Remington, 1979). Considerable evidence supports a major role for products of sensitized T lymphocytes, particularly IFN-γ, in this process. This is especially so in those infections characterized by direct parasitization of macrophages and those in which macrophages play an important role in the host response.

For example, it has long been known that in mice, resistance to listeria infection depends upon the activation of macrophages and that passive protection could be obtained only by transfer of viable peritoneal exudate cells from immune animals (Mackaness, 1964). More recently it has been shown that processing of listeria antigens by macrophages is required for induction of specific T cell immunity (Allen *et al.*, 1984). In the case of infections with *M. avium-intracellulare*, histopathological studies have shown a histiocytic process with a poorly formed or absent granulomata. Acid-fast stains reveal large clusters of mycobacteria ("globi") within tissue histiocytes that have been likened to those observed in another mycobacterial disease, the lepromatous form of leprosy (Macher, 1984). In the latter disease, Nogueira *et al.* (1983) reported a selective defect in the production of IFN-γ by peripheral blood leukocytes in response to specific stimulation with the *M. leprae* antigen and hypothesized that this defect, which could be restored by the addition *in vitro* of interleukin-2, might account for the lack of local macrophage activation in the lepromatous lesions, thereby providing "a fertile intracellular milieu for the uncontrolled replication of the bacilli". By contrast, patients with the tuberculoid form of leprosy, which is commonly a self-limited disease, show normal production of IFN-γ upon challenge with *M. leprae* and have skin lesions characterized by organized granulomata, many helper T cells and scarce or absent live mycobacteria. *T. gondii* is another intracellular pathogen that can replicate freely in normal human and murine mononuclear phagocytes (Murray *et al.*, 1979; Nathan *et al.*, 1983). The addition of natural or recombinant human IFN-γ increased both oxidative metabolism and the killing of *T. gondii* in cultures of human macrophages (Nathan *et al.*, 1983). Pretreatment of mice with murine IFN-γ has been reported to decrease mortality from *T. gondii* (McCabe *et al.*, 1984) and to suppress the replication of *L. monocytogenes* in the spleen (Kiderlen *et al.*, 1984). *P. carinii*, among the most common causes of opportunistic infection in AIDS patients, while not strictly an intracellular pathogen, appears to require intact macrophage function for its control. Rat alveolar and peritoneal macrophages have been shown to ingest and kill *P. carinii in vitro*, although a requirement for opsonizing antibody in this process is controversial (Masur and Jones, 1978; von Behren and Pesanti, 1978). In rats with corticosteroid-induced *P. carinii* pneumonia, Yoneda and Walzer (1980) reported that upon withdrawal of immunosuppressive treatment, clearance of organisms from the lungs coincided with an increase in the number of alveolar macrophages and their ingestion of *P. carinii* cysts. In recent studies of human pulmonary cell populations obtained by bronchoalveolar lavage, a decrease in the proportion (but not the absolute number) of macrophages and an increase in both the proportions and absolute numbers of lymphocytes and polymorphonuclear leukocytes was observed in AIDS patients compared to controls (White *et al.*, 1985; Young *et al.*, 1985). The increase in total lymphocyte numbers was a consequence of increased numbers of OKT8 (Leu 2)-positive cells (Gellene *et al.*, 1984; Wallace *et al.*, 1984; Young *et al.*, 1985). Preliminary data suggest that these changes in pulmonary cell populations precede the development of clinically apparent infection (Young *et al.*, 1985).

All of these observations suggest that a defect in the production of IFN-γ in AIDS patients might account for the frequent occurrence of severe infections that require activated macrophages for their control. Such a defect was first identified by Murray *et al.* (1984), who found that peripheral blood mononuclear cells from AIDS patients who were seropositive to *T. gondii* or had extensive mucosal candidiasis, failed to proliferate or to generate IFN-γ when stimulated with toxoplasma or *C. albicans* antigens respectively. The mononuclear phagocytes of the same patients functioned normally and, when stimulated with IFN-γ, were able to kill *T. gondii*. Lack of proliferation of both unfractionated lymphocytes and purified T4 cells was also observed after stimulation with the soluble protein antigen tetanus toxoid (Lane *et al.*, 1985); however, IFN-γ production was not measured in these experiments.

In yet another study, lymphocytes from 25 of 39 AIDS patients produced no interferon in response to CMV antigen (Epstein *et al.*, 1985). That the stage of disease may influence the capacity of lymphocytes to produce interferon was suggested by the observation that only 3 of 16 patients with opportunistic infection secreted detectable amounts of interferon, whereas interferon was secreted by the lymphocytes of 11 of 23 patients in whom Kaposi's sarcoma was the only manifestation of AIDS. Whether defects in interferon production underlie the predisposition of AIDS patients to CMV infection is uncertain, however, since CMV was isolated from most patients with the chronic lymphadenopathy syndrome in the absence of a defect in interferon production. Furthermore, the presence of CMV viraemia in AIDS patients did not correlate with the level of reduction in the interferon response to CMV stimulation (Epstein *et al.*, 1985).

The observation by Heagy *et al.* (1984) that monocytes from AIDS patients are deficient in their expression of HLA-DR antigens and that normal expression of class II antigens can be induced by incubation of monocytes from AIDS patients with IFN-γ, supports the concept that deficient production of IFN-γ is the proximate cause of the abnormal T cell response to antigen. These authors have speculated that a progressive deficit in T cell production of IL-2 may culminate in a failure to elaborate IFN-γ which, in turn, may account for the low level of class II antigen expression on monocytes. As class-II-positive accessory cells are required for effective antigen presentation to T cells, a vicious cycle can be envisioned, with a progressive decline in both T cell responses to antigens and lymphokine secretion (Heagy *et al.*, 1984). Although this hypothesis has appeal, Rook *et al.* (1985) have shown that the addition of IL-2 to peripheral blood leukocytes from AIDS patients significantly enhanced NK cell activity while failing, in most cases, to induce the release of IFN-γ. In another study, however, Palladino and Welte (1984) showed partial correction of the defect in IFN-γ production when IL-2 was added to lymphocyte cultures. Further support for an IFN-γ-independent mechanism comes from experiments showing that the addition of antibodies to IFN-γ had no effect on IL-2-mediated enhancement of NK activity. Although IFN-γ was itself able to boost NK cell activity, the kinetics of NK cell boosting differed significantly from that induced by IL-2, suggesting independent mechanisms on NK cell activation (Rook *et al.*, 1985).

Deficiencies of IFN-γ production have been observed less consistently after mitogen stimulation. Upon stimulation with concanavalin A (Con A), Murray *et al.* (1984) observed a marked impairment in IFN-γ production in 11 of 16 advanced AIDS patients. The magnitude of the interferon response to Con A was not, however, clearly correlated with lymphocyte numbers or their proliferative response. A similar defect in the IFN-γ response to Con A has been reported by Rook *et al.* (1985). Somewhat different findings were reported by Lane *et al.* (1985), who studied 12 patients who were apparently at an earlier phase in the clinical spectrum of AIDS than those in the previous investigations, and found essentially normal proliferative responses and production of IFN-γ in purified populations of T4 or T8 cells stimulated with pokeweed mitogen (PWM). In addition, whereas the proliferative response of unfractionated mononuclear cells to PWM was diminished, the production of IFN-γ was unimpaired. In neither of these studies was there evidence for active suppression of lymphocyte proliferation or interferon production nor was there evidence for secretion of an inhibitor of IFN-γ.

The findings of Lane *et al.* were corroborated by Epstein *et al.* (1985) who detected interferon production in response to Con A by the lymphocytes of 39 of 40 AIDS patients, with no significant differences in mean titre compared to healthy homosexual and heterosexual controls. However, the lymphocytes of AIDS patients with opportunistic infections produced significantly less interferon than those from patients having Kaposi's sarcoma alone. It is not clear whether the differences observed between these studies can be explained solely on the basis of quantitative differences in the number of T lymphocytes or the effects of repeated opportunistic infections. The finding that an inactivated feline retrovirus (FeLV) markedly inhibits IFN-γ production in cultures of normal feline lymphocytes stimulated with Staphylococcus enterotoxin A, without affecting lymphocyte numbers or viability (Engelman *et al.*, 1985), suggests the possibility that a direct retroviral effect on interferon synthesis, rather than simple reduction in the number of cells capable of synthesizing interferon, may explain the deficient production of IFN-γ in patients with AIDS. Whatever the explanation, the findings support a potential therapeutic role for IFN-γ, either alone or in combination with IL-2, in at least some subsets of AIDS patients.

B Production of an "Aberrant" Interferon

At the same time that some investigators were exploring the possibility that the disordered immune functions and disease susceptibility of AIDS patients were associated with *deficient* interferon production, others were investigating the converse—that abnormal immune function and other AIDS-associated signs and symptoms were related to *excessive* interferon production. Reasoning that many of the immunological abnormalities in AIDS patients, including abnormal T cell subset ratios, polyclonal hyperglobulinaemia and high levels of circulating immune complexes, were reminiscent of those observed in classic autoimmune diseases such as systemic lupus erythematosus (SLE), in which an unusual form of acid-labile IFN-α had been found in the circulation (Skurkovich and Eremkina, 1975; Hooks *et al.*, 1979, 1982; Preble *et al.*, 1982), screening of the serum of AIDS patients and appropriate control populations for the presence of interferon activity was undertaken.

In the first study of this kind, De Stefano *et al.* (1982) found interferon in the serum of 17 (63%) of 27 homosexual men with Kaposi's sarcoma and 10 (29%) of 35 with unexplained generalized lymphadenopathy. Only 2 (8%) of 25 asymptomatic homosexual men and none of 22 heterosexual controls were positive for interferon. As in SLE, the antiviral activity in the serum was similar in tests on human and bovine cells, was specifically neutralized by antibody to human IFN-α, and was inactivated, in most samples, after treatment at pH2 (De Stefano *et al.*, 1982). These results were confirmed in a larger series, which included several patients with AIDS acquired through transfusions of blood or lyophilized clotting factor concentrates (Preble *et al.*, 1984). Hersh *et al.* (1984), while confirming the high frequency of circulating interferon in patients with established AIDS, failed to detect interferon in the serum of 66 homosexual men who were either symptom-free or had the AIDS-related complex. They inferred that the appearance of interferon in the circulation is a late event in AIDS, unrelated to the aetiology of the disease or its manifestations. It has been suggested by others, however, that the presence of acid-labile IFN-α in the serum of otherwise healthy patients in high-risk groups might be a marker for the subsequent development of AIDS, since some haemophiliacs (Eyster *et al.*, 1983) and apparently healthy homosexual men (Buimovici-Klein *et al.*, 1983) who later developed the syndrome were found to have circulating interferon activity that antedated the onset of clinical disease by 2–17 months.

Indirect evidence that the interferon species detected in the serum of AIDS patients is biologically active *in vivo* comes from studies showing abnormally high levels of 2′-5′-oligoadenylate (2-5A) synthetase, an enzyme specifically induced by interferon, in peripheral blood mononuclear cells (Preble *et al.*, 1985), and ultrastructural studies showing the presence of tuboreticular inclusions (TRI) in circulating mononuclear leukocytes (Grimley *et al.*, 1984). Leukocyte TRI have also been observed in various virus infections and in patients with SLE (Baringer, 1971; Gyorkey *et al.*, 1972) and considerable evidence supports a direct role for interferon in their development (Grimley *et al.*, 1983; Rich, 1981). It must be mentioned that the presence or actual levels of serum interferon were not correlated with 2-5A synthetase activity or the frequency of TRI. It is conceivable, however, that local production of interferon in tissues may induce such changes in the absence of detectable serum interferon activity. It is also possible that the elevated serum levels of β_2 microglobulin observed in AIDS patients (Bhalla *et al.*, 1983; Vadhan-Raj *et al.*, 1986a) may reflect the production *in vivo* of interferon. However, the frequency of elevated β_2 microglobulin levels (over 90%) exceeds that of circulating IFN-α activity (Vadhan-Raj *et al.*, 1986a), and the increased levels may simply represent a nonspecific response associated with increased rates of cell membrane turnover. Preble *et al.* (1985) also found that lymphocyte 2-5A synthetase levels failed to increase after systemic treatment or incubation *in vitro* with IFN-α. This contrasts with the observation in normal individuals with viral infections in whom elevated 2-5A synthetase levels could be further increased by incubation with interferon *in vitro* (Penn and Williams, 1984). Although the reason for the decreased synthetase induction by exogenous interferon in AIDS patients is unclear, several hypotheses have been proposed, including depression of interferon receptors, induction of a nonfunctional enzyme, or the presence of inhibitors of 2-5A synthetase activity.

It is conceivable that many of the nonspecific signs and symptoms seen in patients with AIDS and the AIDS-related complex also reflect the presence of interferon production *in vivo*. Unexplained fever, in the absence of documented infection, is common in AIDS and is a well described side-effect of treatment with exogenous interferons. Similarly, malaise, fatigue, anorexia, weight loss and neutropenia in the absence of a hypocellular bone marrow are common both in AIDS patients and those receiving treatment with interferon for other conditions. Although other explanations for these signs and symptoms are possible, considerable evidence points to a direct role for interferon in mediating the pathology associated with certain viral and autoimmune diseases in humans and experimental animals (reviewed in Vilček, 1984). Stronger support for a direct role for interferon in the pathogenesis of some of the manifestations of AIDS would require studies showing a correlation between the presence of circulating interferon and the occurrence of AIDS symptoms. If such a correlation could be shown, it would follow that attempts to remove or inactivate interferon in the circulation might ameliorate some of the symptoms (and, perhaps, some of the immunological abnormalities) in AIDS patients, a possibility that has been raised by Vilček (1984). Metroka *et al.* (1984) have, indeed, suggested that serum antiviral titres may correlate with the severity of certain systemic symptoms, although quantitative data were not given in their report.

The nature of the inducer, the cellular source and the biological significance of the circulating IFN-α activity found in AIDS patients is unknown. Although NK cells have been shown to produce an acid-labile IFN-α in response to tumour cells (Trinchieri *et al.*, 1979), the fact that interferon activity is present in AIDS patients and high-risk individuals without Kaposi's sarcoma, but is absent in patients with traditional African Kaposi's sarcoma (Preble *et al.*, 1984; Eglin *et al.*, 1984), makes it unlikely that Kaposi's sarcoma cells are the stimulus for interferon production in AIDS. It is known that lymphocytes from normal individuals vaccinated against influenza produce acid-labile IFN-α when stimulated *in vitro* with influenza virus (Balkwill *et al.*, 1983) and, prior to the discovery of HTLV-III, considerable speculation centred on the role of persistent virus infection, particularly with CMV, as the stimulus for interferon production in AIDS. However, attempts to correlate the presence of CMV infection with that of endogenous interferon were generally unsuccessful (De Stefano *et al.*, 1982). More recent studies indicate that B cell lines established from patients with AIDS secrete large amounts of acid-labile IFN-α and harbour HTLV-III (C. Metroka, personal communication). In a multivariate analysis of immunological variables as potential prognostic factors, our group has shown that the presence of acid-labile serum interferon activity was the single most important predictor of survival in patients with Kaposi's sarcoma and AIDS (Vadhan-Raj *et al.*, 1986a). At the time of our analysis, only 26% of patients who had circulating interferon activity when first evaluated were alive, whereas the survival rate was 73% in those in whom interferon was absent. These data, and others showing the importance of **B** cell functional tests in predicting prognosis (Vadhan-Raj *et al.*, 1986a), support one possibility—that HTLV-III is the inducer, and the infected B cell the source of the observed interferon activity. Further study will, of course, be required to evaluate this hypothesis.

Recently reported findings by Birx *et al.*, (1986) in patients with AIDS and related disorders suggest that infection of B cells with Epstein-Barr virus (EBV) may be an alternative explanation for the high frequency of circulating IFN-α activity. Such patients were shown to have defective *in vitro* T-cell regulation of EBV-infected B cells as well as abnormally high numbers of EBV-infected B cells in the circulation. In this study, no evidence was found for coinfection of the EBV-transformed B cell clones with HTLV-III. However, the ability of HTLV-III/LAV to infect EBV-positive B cells *in vitro* has been previously demonstrated (Montaigner *et al.*, 1984), and coinfection of B cells with both viruses *in vivo* cannot be excluded as a possibility.

In his essay, "The Importance of Having Gamma", Jan Vilček describes a meeting during which the idea for examining the serum of Kaposi's sarcoma patients for interferon was first proposed (Vilček, 1982). The possibility was raised that antibodies detected on the surface of lymphocytes in AIDS patients might, in much the same way as OKT3 monoclonal antibodies, induce the production of IFN-γ. Although most reports have failed to substantiate this hypothesis, two of the patients reported by Buimovici-Klein (1983) did, in fact, have IFN-γ rather than IFN-α activity in the serum. Furthermore, IL-2 stimulated T cells from patients with AIDS have been reported to spontaneously generate IFN-γ in culture (Moore *et al.*, 1985). It is, perhaps, conceivable that the short serum half-life of IFN-γ may have prevented its detection in larger numbers of patients, or that depletion of the T cell pool resulted in only a transient IFN-γ response.

III INTERFERON AS TREATMENT

> . . . if interferon is responsible for some of the disease symptoms, attempts to use it for the treatment of AIDS will only add insult to injury. . . Jan Vilček (1984).

A Kaposi's Sarcoma

I quote Professor Vilček's remark with tongue firmly planted in cheek, coming as it did some time after the demonstration by our group (Krown *et al.*, 1983) that some patients with AIDS-associated Kaposi's sarcoma could, in fact, derive benefit from treatment with IFN-α. His remark does, of course, underscore an important dilemma in our understanding of the mechanisms underlying tumour development? Or are we, perhaps, also seeing When tumour regression is observed, are we simply seeing the result of a direct antiproliferative effect on tumour cells that has no bearing on the mechanisms underlying tumour development? Or are we, perhaps, also seeing a result mediated through interferon-induced effects on host defences or virus proliferation that may have direct bearing on the pathogenesis of the tumour? Is interferon a treatment for AIDS itself or merely for an epiphenomenon of the syndrome? These questions cannot be answered with certainty, as the data thus far can be interpreted as supporting either hypothesis.

The first demonstration that IFN-α could induce the regression of Kaposi's sarcoma occurred in the last quarter of 1981, probably the most exciting but frenetic few months of my life. Earlier that year I had begun a Phase I study of a recombinant IFN-α preparation (Clone A) from Hoffmann-La Roche (then abbreviated IFL-rA, subsequently abbreviated rIFN-αA, and currently going by the name of IFN-α2a or Roferon-A). Together with Francisco X. (Paco) Real, a new and enthusiastic fellow recently arrived from Barcelona, we treated cancer patients at various increasing dosage levels, and had reached a dose of 36 million units by late summer. In mid-September a 32-year-old man with Kaposi's sarcoma involving the skin, lymph nodes, hard palate and gastrointestinal tract was referred to me by Bijan Safai, the head of our Dermatology Service, who had long maintained an investigative interest in this tumour. The patient began treatment on 29 September and within four weeks had shown marked regression of his oral and cutaneous tumours. Two more patients with Kaposi's sarcoma were started on treatment in October. In early November I briefly disappeared from this exciting scene, gave birth to a daughter, and returned to work (after what some of my less sensitive colleagues referred to as my "vacation") on 30 November, by which time five Kaposi's sarcoma patients were already on study. Three more patients began treatment by year's end, and five more by February of 1982, comprising the 13 patients described in our 1983 report (Krown *et al.*, 1983). Of that group, three showed complete disappearance of their tumours and two showed partial (over 50%) tumour regression, an overall major response rate of 38%. This represented the first demonstration that a pure, single species of IFN-α had activity against a specific tumour type. In fact, our study and others that followed have shown Kaposi's sarcoma to be the non-lymphohaematopoietic malignancy that is most consistently responsive to IFN-α treatment.

A summary of various published therapeutic trials with different, highly purified IFN-α preparations (including alpha-2a, alpha-2b and lymphoblastoid interferons) is given in Table I. The studies, although varying somewhat in specific details of route and schedule of drug administration, are similar in their conclusions. When given in sufficiently high doses, highly purified alpha interferons are capable of inducing tumour regression in a substantial proportion of patients with Kaposi's sarcoma, with a mean response rate of approximately 30% (61 of 201) in patients treated at doses of at least 20

TABLE I Interferon α Trials in Kaposi's Sarcoma

IFN species	Dose ($\times 10^{-6}$ U)	Route[a]	Schedule	Major Responses[b]	Reference
alfa-2a	36[c]	IM	Daily	13/34 (38)	Krown *et al.* (1983) Krown *et al.* (1984) Real *et al.* (1986a)
	3	IM	Daily	1/36 (3)	Krown *et al.* (1984) Real *et al.* (1986a)
	3 → 36[d] (in low dose failures)	IM	Daily	5/30 (17)	Krown *et al.* (1984) Real *et al.* (1986a)
	3 → 36 (as initial treatment)	IM	Daily	4/27 (15)	Real *et al.* (1986b)
alfa-2b	$50/m^2$	IV	Daily × 5 every other week	4/10 (40)	Groopman *et al.* (1984)
	$1/m^2$	SC	Daily × 5 every other week	2/10 (20)	Groopman *et al.* (1984)
	1 → $50/m^2$ (in low dose failures)	IV	Daily × 5 every other week	2/4 (50)	Groopman *et al.* (1984)
	$50/m^2$	IV	Daily × 5 every other week	8/20 (40)	Volberding *et al.* (1984a)
	$30/m^2$	SC	Three times per week	14/56 (25)	Mitsuyasu *et al.* (1984)
alfa-Ly	$20/m^2$	IM	Daily	8/12 (67)	Rios *et al.* (1985a)
	$7.5/m^2$	IM	Daily	1/9 (67)	Gelmann *et al.* (1985)
	$15/m^2$	IM	Daily	0/10 (0)	Gelmann *et al.* (1985)
	$25/m^2$	IM	Daily	3/8 (38)	Gelmann *et al.* (1985)

[a] IM, intramuscular; IV, intravenous; SC, subcutaneous.
[b] Number of complete or partial responses/Number of evaluable patients (percent major responses).
[c] Three patients began treatment at a dose of 54×10^6 U/day.
[d] → Signifies dose escalation from the lower to the higher dose shown.

million units per square metre body surface area. Patients treated with lower doses responded infrequently, however, with an overall response rate of 6% (4 of 65 patients, $p < 0.001$). The difference in response rates between high- and low-dose regimens has been interpreted by some as signifying a direct antiproliferative action of interferon on the tumour. An alternative explanation may be that higher doses of interferon are required to stimulate host defence mechanisms or to inhibit virus replication, a hypothesis that, unfortunately, has not yet been subjected to formal testing.

Considerable progress has been made in identifying prognostic factors that correlate with responsiveness to the antitumour effects of interferon. Although Rios *et al.* (1985a) suggested that the very high response rate (67%) observed in a preliminary study of human lymphoblastoid interferon might be related to the preponderance of patients with minimal tumour burden in that trial, our analysis of a much larger group of patients showed no significant association between response to treatment and either tumour burden or the presence of gastrointestinal involvement (Real *et al.*, 1986a). The indirect evidence suggesting a multicentric origin of Kaposi's sarcoma (Templeton, 1981; Costa and Rabson, 1983) supports the concept that gastrointestinal tract involvement with Kaposi's sarcoma does not have the same negative prognostic significance as visceral metastases in other tumour types.

A history of opportunistic infection has consistently been associated with a poor response to subsequent interferon treatment (Krown *et al.*, 1984; Mitsuyasu *et al.*, 1984; Gelmann *et al.*, 1985; Real *et al.*, 1986a). Similarly, the presence of unexplained fevers or weight loss (so-called "B" symptoms) has been associated with lack of responsiveness to interferon, although in at least one reported patient, complete tumour regression was associated with resolution of such systemic symptoms (Groopman *et al.*, 1984). Such observations suggest that the severity of clinical symptoms may directly reflect the degree of immunological impairment in patients with Kaposi's sarcoma, a possibility also suggested by Volberding *et al.* (1984b), who found that the severity of anaemia and the number of "B" symptoms were the most important clinical factors associated with survival.

Although the lack of consistent improvement in immune function in patients receiving interferon as treatment for Kaposi's sarcoma has supported arguments against a role for IFN-α in the treatment of AIDS-associated immune deficiency, considerable evidence suggests that relative preservation of immune function is required for interferon to be active as an antitumour agent. Several studies have now confirmed that the presence of acid-labile IFN-α in the serum prior to treatment is associated with lack of responsiveness to exogenous IFN-α (Krown *et al.*, 1984; Gelmann *et al.*, 1985; Rios *et al.*, 1985a; Vadhan-Raj *et al.*, 1986a). Although it has been speculated that the low rate of tumour response in such patients may reflect a state of resistance to interferon's effects (Gelmann *et al.*, 1985), in our experience the presence of endogenous interferon was not associated with reduced responsiveness to augmentation of natural killer cell cytotoxicity by interferon *in vitro* (Vadhan-Raj *et al.*, 1986a). Others have, however, reported that incubation with IFN-α (Reddy *et al.*, 1984) or IFN-β (Rook *et al.*, 1983) failed to augment natural killer cell cytotoxicity of peripheral blood mononuclear cells from patients with more severe infectious complications of AIDS than those included in our study.

Other measures of immune cell numbers or functions have also been correlated with interferon responsiveness. Gelmann *et al.* (1985) found a significant association between response and total numbers of lymphocytes and OKT4+ cells in the circulation. In an analysis of 20 immunological variables, Vadhan-Raj *et al.* (1986a) found that high lymphoproliferative responses to microbial activators (believed to function as B cell mitogens) and preservation of delayed hypersensitivity responses to one or more recall antigens were significantly associated with response to interferon. In a logistic regression model, patients with positive delayed type hypersensitivity reactions and relatively high proliferative responses to an *E. coli* antigen preparation were predicted to have a 75% response rate to interferon, whereas those who were anergic and had low lymphoproliferative responses had a predicted response rate of 9.5%. The observed response rates—70% and 12.5%, respectively—were close to those predicted by the model (Vadhan-Raj *et al.*, 1986a). The association of tumour regression with the status of immune function by no means establishes the mechanism by which interferon induces its antitumour effects. On the other hand, there is no reason to think that relative preservation of immune function should be associated with tumour regression if the sole mechanism is a direct antiproliferative one. It is of interest in this context that the ability of IFN-α to augment 2-5A synthetase levels, considered an index of biological responsiveness to interferon, was inconsistent in patients with Kaposi's sarcoma and failed to correlate with the clinical response (Preble *et al.*, 1985).

Although oncologists and their patients are always delighted to observe tumour regression, the true test of a treatment regimen is its impact on the quality and duration of patient survival. This is particularly so in AIDS-associated Kaposi's sarcoma, a tumour which, while producing significant morbidity in some individuals, is only infrequently a direct cause of death. In a long-term follow-up study of patients treated with recombinant interferon alpha-2a, those whose tumours regressed showed a highly significant reduction in the number of subsequent opportunistic infections and longer survival compared to those whose tumours did not respond (Real *et al.*, 1986a). However, it cannot be determined whether these differences reflect an effect of interferon on the natural history of the disease or a higher response rate of patients whose disease takes a more favourable course for other reasons. Drug tolerability is another important factor in assessing the value of treatment. Although some patients, particularly those treated at high doses, have required reduction of the interferon dose, most commonly because of severe fatigue and less often because of hypotension, elevation of hepatic transaminases or lowering of the white blood cell count, most studies have indicated that IFN-α is relatively well tolerated in the large majority of such patients. In our own experience, patients with Kaposi's sarcoma tolerated treatment better and required dose reduction less often than those with renal cell carcinoma treated at the same interferon dose and schedule.

A number of questions remain to be answered concerning the optimal use of IFN-α in Kaposi's sarcoma. In responding patients, the optimal duration of treatment is unknown. In the past, our practice had been to discontinue treatment one month after confirmation of complete tumour regression. Although several patients remain in unmaintained remission for periods of one to two years, others developed tumour recurrence after interferon treatment was stopped. In our limited experience with such patients, response to a second course of interferon treatment has been less successful (Real *et al.*, 1986a). Our current practice is to continue treatment indefinitely in responding patients, but it is premature to say whether this will result in more durable responses.

The role of IFN-α in combination with other treatments has yet to be adequately investigated. Although Rios *et al.* (1985b) have suggested an improved response rate in patients treated with a combination of lymphoblastoid interferon and vinblastine, a preliminary randomized trial comparing interferon alpha-2a alone or in combination with vinblastine has shown no difference in response rates (Krown *et al.* 1986). In the latter study, most patients receiving combination therapy developed unacceptable haematological toxicity, precluding administration of the planned vinblastine doses. Other combinations, particularly with immunologically active agents (IL-2 or IFN-γ, for example) have yet to be explored.

Finally, a few words about IFN-γ are in order. Despite the data indicating deficient production of this lymphokine in AIDS patients, scarce supplies have, until quite recently, precluded the clinical investigations logically suggested by these observations. Several years ago, Odajnyk *et al.* (1984) reported on the results in seven patients treated with a human IFN-γ preparation. All showed progression of Kaposi's sarcoma and three reportedly had rapid progression of previously stable disease. The results of this study are difficult to interpret, however, given the small sample size and the known contamination of the interferon preparation with other biologically active cytokines. More recently, with the availability of highly purified recombinant IFN-γ preparations, additional patients have been treated, although published reports are scarce. In a Phase I trial of recombinant IFN-γ we included five patients with Kaposi's sarcoma who were treated with intravenous infusions over a dose range of 0.1–1.0 mg/m^2 ($\sim$2–20 $\times$ 10^6 U/m^2). Although a reduction in the size of enlarged lymph nodes was observed in one patient, there were no major antitumour responses and no improvement in T cell numbers or subset ratios (Vadhan-Raj *et al.*, 1986b). Our impression was that these patients experienced somewhat more severe constitutional and haematological toxicity than other cancer patients without AIDS, an observation that may be explained by the co-existence of endogenous acid-labile IFN-α in the circulation of four of the five patients. The preliminary indication that IFN-γ lacks efficacy against Kaposi's sarcoma does not, however, exclude a role for this agent in the treatment or prevention of some of the other manifestations of AIDS. Carl Nathan and his group have shown that treatment of cancer patients with quite low and well-tolerated doses of recombinant IFN-γ significantly increases the hydrogen peroxide secretory capacity of circulating monocytes (Nathan *et al.*, 1985), a finding recently confirmed in patients with lepromatous leprosy using even lower interferon doses (C. F. Nathan, personal communication). Thus, while apparently not active against the major neoplastic complication of AIDS, IFN-γ may offer a means of dealing with some of the more deadly infectious complications of the syndrome.

B AIDS-associated Infections

A potential role for IFN-γ in the treatment of various opportunistic infections is currently at the stage of hopeful speculation. The news is less encouraging for IFN-α. As discussed previously, the low rate of opportunistic infection in patients whose tumours respond to IFN-α is heartening, but may have little to do with the interferon treatment itself. On the other hand, Gelmann *et al.* (1985) showed no effect of lymphoblastoid interferon treatment on CMV recovery from patients with Kaposi's sarcoma, and some of their patients developed new sites of CMV infection during or immediately after interferon therapy. Using moderate to high doses of partially purified human alpha (leukocyte) interferon, Chou *et al.* (1984) detected no significant effect in four patients with CMV retinitis, three of whom had AIDS. Viruria increased during treatment in two of the AIDS patients, and both developed total blindness. The lack of efficacy of interferon in established CMV infection should come as no major surprise, since even in those infections known to be affected by interferon, prophylaxis or early therapy is more beneficial than treatment late in the course of the disease (Pazin *et al.*, 1979; Hirsch *et al.*, 1983; Merigan *et al.*, 1982). The basis for interferon's lack of efficacy has been suggested by the results of a preliminary study of AIDS patients with positive CMV cultures in which IL-2 was shown to augment NK cell and CMV-specific lymphocyte cytotoxic activities *in vitro*, but IFN-β had little or no effect (Rook *et al.*, 1983). The ability of interferons to prevent or ameliorate the course of other AIDS-associated infections has not been formally investigated.

C Immune Deficiency

There are currently little data to support a role for IFN-α alone in the treatment of AIDS-associated immune deficiency. Although our preliminary study suggested that interferon treatment was associated with modest augmentation in peripheral blood natural killer cell activity, the lymphoproliferative response to PHA stimulation and the OKT4+/OKT8+ ratio (Krown *et al.*, 1983), our subsequent analyses of a larger number of patients have shown inconsistent changes that correlate poorly with therapeutic response. Groopman *et al.* (1984) also found an increase in natural killer cell activity in some interferon-treated patients, but noted a significant decline in the ratio of helper (Leu-3+) to suppressor (Leu-2+) cells. Rios *et al.* (1985a) found no significant change in NK cell activity during four weeks of treatment with lymphoblastoid interferon, but observed a progressive decline in the total number of lymphocytes, individual lymphocyte subsets, lymphocyte blastogenic responses to mitogens, ADCC and the number of adherent monocytes in the circulation. It must be emphasized that these data come from preliminary trials in small numbers of patients who were followed over a relatively brief period of treatment. With larger numbers of patients and longer follow-up it may yet be possible to discern effects of interferon treatment on immune function and to correlate such effects with antitumour activity.

D HTLV-III

One of the initial reasons for considering the use of interferon in patients with AIDS was to treat a tumour in which a virus was believed to play some aetiological role. Although it turned out that the virus selected as the target of the attack, CMV, was probably the wrong one, the right agent may have been chosen. Interferon alpha-2a has recently been shown to have a dose-related suppressive effect on HTLV-III replication in normal peripheral blood mononuclear cells. Inhibition occurred at concentrations that were both non-toxic to the target cells in culture and which can be achieved in the blood after intramuscular injection (Ho *et al.*, 1985). Subsequent unpublished studies by Martin Hirsch and his colleagues in Boston have shown interferon alpha-2a to be superior to interferons alfa-D and beta in its ability to inhibit HTLV-III replication, while IFN-γ had no activity against the virus.

The recent development of techniques to culture HTLV-III from the blood of patients with AIDS and those in high-risk groups now permits prospective studies to evaluate the effects *in vivo* of IFN-α treatment on the aetiological agent and to define the stage of infection at which such treatment might be of greatest benefit. Although the precise mechanisms of IFN-α's anti-HTLV-III effects are not known, its effects on animal retroviruses are believed to be mediated in part by alterations in virus assembly or release—i.e. at a late stage of virus replication. This raises the possibility of combining IFN-α with other agents that exert their antiviral effects by different mechanisms, for example inhibitors of reverse transcriptase, in order to seek evidence of synergistic antiviral effects.

IV CONCLUDING REMARKS

The acquired immunodeficiency syndrome has two sides. On the one hand it has been characterized as a modern-day plague, inducing untold despair, suffering and death. On the other, the disease offers potential bonuses. It teaches us about human needs, about fear, about caring and compassion. It provides a unique opportunity to study the role of viruses and the immune system in tumour development. It gives us a means of understanding the normal functioning of the immune system through study of its pathology. And, as I have tried to review here, it is teaching us a good deal about the interferon system and its role in the pathogenesis and treatment of disease.

In the epilogue to his 1982 essay in this series. Vilček suggests that had Pygmalion been a biomedical scientist, he might have created interferon—a substance with virtues "almost too splendid to be true"—to be his Galatea. I would suggest that had Robert Louis Stevenson been an AIDS researcher of philosophical nature seeking an appropriate metaphor for the coexistence of good and evil, he might also have chosen interferon. For, like the character of Dr Jekyll and Mr Hyde, interferon, while certainly possessing great virtues, has a dark and sinister side. That, of course, only adds to its fascination.

ACKNOWLEDGEMENTS

The care and study of patients with AIDS requires the coordinated and dedicated efforts of many individuals. The clinical studies performed at this Center and cited here could not have been carried out without the active participation and support of the fellows, research nurses and data management staff of the Clinical Immunology Service and numerous collaborators in the laboratories of the Sloan-Kettering Institute. The contribution of two individuals is particularly acknowledged—Paco Real, who has shared fully in the sometimes overwhelming responsibilities for patient care and treatment and Saroj Vadhan-Raj who, together with members of our biostatistics group, transformed a huge body of immunological data into a form that gives useful information about prognosis, appropriate treatment strategies and possible clues to the role of interferon in the disease process. I thank Pamela Webster for preparing the many revisions of this manuscript and Hoffmann-La Roche Inc. and NIH grants CA-33049 and CA-34995 for support of this work.

REFERENCES

Abb, J., Kochen, M. and Deinhardt, F. (1984). *Infection* **12**, 240–242.

Allen, P. M., Beller, D. I., Braun, J. and Unanue, E. R. (1984). *J. Immunol.* **132**, 323–331.

Balkwill, F. R., Griffin, D. B., Band, H. A. and Beverly, P. C. L. (1983). *J. Exp. Med.* **157**, 1059–1063.

Barré-Sinoussi, F., Chermann, J. C., Rey, F., Nugeyre, M. T., Chamaret, S., Gruest, J., Dauguet, C. and Axler-Blin, C. (1983). *Science* **220**, 868–871.

Baringer, J. R. (1971). *New. Engl. J. Med.* **285**, 943–945.

Bhalla, R. B., Safai, B., Mertelsmann, R. and Schwartz, M. (1983). *Clin. Chem.* **29**, 1560 (letter).

Birx, D. L., Redfield, R. R. and Tosato, G. (1986). *N. Engl. J. Med.* **314**, 874–879.

Buimovici-Klein, E., Lange, M., Klein, R. J., Cooper, L. Z. and Grieco, M. H. (1983). *Lancet* **2**, 344.

Centers for Disease Control (1981a). *MMWR* **30**, 250–252.

Centers for Disease Control (1981b). *MMWR* **30**, 305–308.

Centers for Disease Control (1982). *MMWR* **31**, 507–514.

Centers for Disease Control (1985) *MMWR* **34**, 373–375.

Chou, S., Dylewski, J. S., Gaynon, M. W., Egbert, P. R. and Merigan, T. C. (1984). *Antimicrob. Agents Chemother.* **25**, 25–28.

Ciobanu, N., Andreef, M., Safai, B. Koziner, B. and Mertelsmann, R. (1983). *Ann. Int. Med.* **98**, 151–155.

Costa, J. and Rabson, A. S. (1983). *Lancet* **1**, 58.

DeStefano, E., Friedman, R. M., Freidman-Kien, A. E., Goedert, J. J., Henriksen, D., Preble, O. T., Sonnabend, J. A. and Vilček, J. (1982). *J. Infect. Dis.* **146**, 451–455.

Eglin, R. P., Kurtz, J. B., and Downing, R. G. (1984). *Lancet* **1**, 564–565.

Engelman, R. W., Fulton, R. W., Good, R. A. and Day, N. K. (1985). *Science* **227**, 1368–1370.

Epstein, E. (1972). *JAMA* **219**, 1477–1478.

Epstein, J. S., Frederick, W. R., Rook, A. H., Jackson, L., Manischewitz, J. F., Mayner, R. E., Masur, H., Enterline, J. C., Djeu, J. Y. and Quinnan, G. V. Jr. (1985). *J. Infect. Dis.* **152**, 727–733.

Eyster, M. E., Goedert, J. J., Poon, M-C. and Preble, O. T. (1983). *New Engl. J. Med.* **309**, 583–586.

Friedman-Kien, A. E., Laubenstein, L. J., Rubenstein, P., Buimovici-Klein, E.,

Marmor, M., Stahl, R., Spigland, I., Kim, K. S., and Zolla-Pazner, S. (1982). *Ann. Int. Med.* **96**, 705–713.

Gallo, R. C., Salahuddin, S. Z., Popovic, M., Shearer, G. M., Kaplan, M., Haynes, B. F., Palker, T. J., Redfield, R., Oleske, J., Safai, B., White, G., Foster, P. and Markham, P. D. (1984). *Science* **224**, 500–503.

Gellene, R. A., Stover, D. E., Gebbard, D., Evans, R. L. and Cunningham-Rundles, C., (1984). *Clin. Res.* **32**, 429A.

Gelmann, E. P., Preble, O. T., Steis, R., Lane, H. C., Rook, A. H., Wesley, M., Jacob, J., Fauci, A., Masur, H. and Longo, D. (1985). *Amer. J. Med.* **78**, 737–741.

Gerstoft, J., Malchow-Møller, A., Bygbjerg, I., Dickmeiss, E., Enk, C., Halberg, P., Haahr, S., Jacobsen, M., Jensen, K., Mejer, J., Nielsen, J. O., Thomsen, H. K., Søndergaard, J. and Lorenzen, I. (1982). *Br. Med. J.* **285**, 17–19.

Giraldo, G., Beth, E. and Haguenau, F. (1972). *J. Natl Cancer Inst.* **49**, 1509–1526.

Giraldo, G., Beth, E., Kaurilsky, F. M., Henle, W., Henle, G., Miké, V., Huraux, J. M., Anderson, M. K., Charbi, M. R., Kyalwazi, S. K. and Puissant, A. (1975). *Int. J. Cancer* **15**, 839–848.

Giraldo, G., Beth, E., Henle, W., Henle, G., Miké, V., Safai, B., Huraux, J. M., McHardy, J. and De Thé, G. (1978). *Int. J. Cancer* **22**, 126–131.

Gottlieb, M. S., Schroff, R., Schanker, H. M., Weisman, J. D., Fain, P. T., Wolf, R. A. and Saxon, A. (1981). *New Engl. J. Med.* **305**, 1425–1431.

Grimley, P. M., Kang, Y-H., Silverman, R. H., Davis, G. and Hoofnagle, J. H. (1983). *Lab. Invest.* **48**, 30A.

Grimley, P. M., Kang, Y-H., Frederick, W., Rook, A. H., Kostianovsky, M., Sonnabend, J. A., Macher, A., Quinnan, G. V., Friedman, R. M. and Masur, H. (1984). *Amer. J. Clin. Pathol.* **81**, 147–155.

Groopman, J. E., Gottlieb, M. S., Goodman, J., Mitsuyasu, R. T., Conant, M. A., Prince, H., Fahey, J. L., Derezin, M., Weinstein, W. M., Casavante, C., Rothman, J., Rudnick, S. A. and Volberding, P. A. (1984). *Ann. Int. Med.* **100**, 671–676.

Gyorkey, F., Sinkovics, J. G., Min, K. W. and Gyorkey, P. (1972). *Amer. J. Med.* **53**, 148.

Hahn, B. H. (1985). *Ann. Int. Med.* **102**, 807–809.

Harwood, A. R., Osaba, D. and Hofstader, S. L., (1979). *Amer. J. Med.* **67**, 759–765.

Heagy, W., Kelley, V. E., Strom, T. B., Mayer, K., Shapiro, H. M., Mandel, R. and Finberg, R. (1984). *J. Clin. Invest.* **74**, 2089–2096.

Hersh, E. M., Mansell, P. W. A., Reuben, J. M., Rios, A. and Newell, G. R. (1984). *Cancer Res.* **44**, 5894–5901.

Hersh, E. M., Gutterman, J. U., Spector, S., Friedman, H., Greenberg, S. B., Reuben, J. M., La Pushin, R., Matza, M. and Mansell, P. W. A. (1985). *Cancer Res.* **45**, 406–410.

Hirsch, M. S., Schooley, R. T. and Cosimi, B., (1983). *New Engl. J. Med.* **308**, 1489–1493.

Ho, D. D., Hartshorn, K. L., Rota, T. R., Andrews, C. A., Kaplan, J. C., Schooley, R. T. and Hirsch, M. S. (1985). *Lancet* **1**, 602–604.

Hooks, J. J., Moutsopoulos, H. M., Geis, S. A., Stahl, N. I., Decker, J. L. and Notkins, A. L. (1979). *New Engl. J. Med.* **301**, 5–8.

Hooks, J. J., Jordan, G. W., Cupps, T., Moutsopoulos, H. M., Fauci, A. S., and Notkins, A. L. (1982). *Arthritis Rheum.* **25**, 396–400.

Ikossi-O'Connor, M. G., Ambrus, J. L., West, T., Lillie, M. A., Milgrom, H. and Chadha, K. C. (1984). *Res. Commun. Chem. Pathol. Pharmacol.* **45**, 271–277.

Kaposi, M. (1872). *Arch. Dermatol. Syph.* **4**, 265–273.
Keen, P. (1962). *Cancer* **18**, 380–387.
Kiderlen, A. F., Kaufmann, S. H. E. and Lohmann-Matthes, M.-L. (1984). *Eur J. Immunol.* **14**, 964–967.
Klein, M. B., Pereira, F. A. and Kantor, I. (1974). *Arch. Dermatol.* **110**, 602–604.
Krown, S. E. (1984). *J. Psychosoc. Oncol.* **2**, 1–17.
Krown, S. E., Real, F. X., Cunningham-Rundles, S., Myskowski, P. L., Koziner, B., Fein, S., Mittleman, A., Oettgen, H. F. and Safai, B. (1983). *New Eng. J. Med.* **308**, 1071–1076.
Krown, S. E., Real, F. X., Krim, M., Cunningham-Rundles, S., Koziner, B., Myskowski, P. L., Safai, B. and Oettgen, H. F. (1984). *Ann. NY Acad. Sci.* **437**, 431–437.
Krown, S. E., Real, F. X., Lester, T. and Oettgen, H. F. (1986). *Proc. Amer. Soc. Clin. Oncol.* **5**, 6.
Lane, H. C., Depper, J. M., Greene, W. C., Whalen, G., Waldmann, T. A. and Fauci, A. (1985). *New Engl. J. Med.* **313**, 79–84.
Longo, D. L. (1984). *Ann. Int. Med.* **100**, 96–98.
Lopez, C., Fitzgerald, P. A. and Siegal, F. P. (1983). *J. Infect. Dis.* **148**, 962–966.
Lopez, C., Fitzgerald, P. A., Siegal, F. P., Landesman, S., Gold, J. and Krown, S. E. (1984). *Ann. NY. Acad. Sci.* **437**, 39–47.
Lothe, F. (1963). *Acta. Pathologica. Microbiol. Scand.* (*Suppl*). **161**, 1–71.
McCabe, R. E., Luft, B. J. and Remington, J. S. (1984). *J. Infect. Dis.* **150**, 961–962.
Macher, A. (1984). *Ann. Int. Med.* **100**, 94–96.
Mackaness, G. B. (1964). *J. Exp. Med.* **120**, 105–120.
Master, S. P., Taylor, J. F., Kyalwazi, S. K. and Ziegler, J. L. (1970). *Br. Med. J.* **1**, 600–602.
Masur, H. and Jones, T. C. (1978). *J. Exp. Med.* **147**, 157–170.
Masur, H., Michelis, M. A., Greene, J. B., Onorato, I, Murray, H. W. and Cunningham-Rundles, S. (1981). *New Engl. J. Med.* **305**, 1431–1438.
Merigan, T. C., Rand, K. H., Pollard, R. B., (1978). *New Engl. J. Med.* **298**, 981–987.
Metroka, C. E., Cunningham-Rundles, S., Pollack, M. S., Sonnabend, J. A., Davis, J. M., Gordon, B., Fernandez, R. D. and Mouradian, J. (1983). *Ann. Int. Med.* **9**, 585–591.
Metroka, C. E., Cunningham-Rundles, S., Krim, M., Pollack, M. S. Sonnabend, J. A., Gunby, T. C., Alonso, M. L., Davis, J. M., Mouradian, J. and Witkin, S. S. (1984). *Ann. NY. Acad. Sci.* **437**, 400–409.
Mitsuyasu, R., Volberding, P., Jacobs, A., Champlin, R., Moran, T., Golando, J., Valero, R. and Spiegel, R. (1984). *Proc. Amer. Soc. Clin. Oncol.* **3**, 51.
Moertel, C. G. (1966). *Recent Results Cancer Res.* **7**, 34–47.
Montaigner, L., Gruest, J., Chamaret, S., Dauguet, C., Axler, C., Guétard, D., Nugeyre, M. T., Barré-Sinoussi, F., Chermann, J.-C., Brunet, J. B., Klatzmann, D. and Gluckman, J. C. (1984). *Science* **225**, 63–66.
Moore, J. L., Poiesz, B. J., Tomar, R. H., Merl, S. A. and Ehrlich, G. D. (1985). *New Engl. J. Med.* **312**, 442–443.
Murray, H. W., Juangbhanich, C. W., Nathan, C. F. and Cohn, Z. A. (1979). *J. Exp. Med.* **150**, 950.
Murray, H. W., Rubin, B. Y., Masur, H. and Roberts, R. B. (1984). *New Engl. J. Med.* **310**, 883–889.
Myers, B. D., Kessler, E., Lepi, J., Pick, A., Rosenfeld, J. B. and Tikvah, P. (1974). *Arch. Int. Med.* **133**, 307–311.

Nathan, C. F., Murray, H. W., Weibe, M. E. and Rubin, B. Y. (1983). *J. Exp. Med.* **158**, 670–689.

Nathan, C. F., Horowitz, C. R., de la Harpe, J., Vadhan-Raj, S., Sherwin, S. A., Oettgen, H. F. and Krown, S. E. (1985). *Proc. Natl. Acad. Sci. USA* **82**, 8686–8690.

Nogueira, N., Kaplan, G., Levy, E., Sarno, E., N., Kushner, P., Granelli-Piperno, A., Vieira, L., Gould, V. C., Levis, W., Steinman, R., Yip, Y. K. and Cohn, Z. A. (1983). *J. Exp. Med.* **158**, 2165–2170.

Odajnyk, C., Laubenstein, L., Friedman-Kien, A., Ostreicher, R., Vilček, J., Rubinstein, P. and Krigel, R. (1984). *Proc. Amer. Soc. Clin. Oncol.* **3**, 61.

Oettle, A. G. (1962). *Acta Un Int Cancer* **18**, 330–363.

Oettle, A. G. (1963). *In* "Symposium on Kaposi's Sarcoma" (L. V. Ackerman and J. F. Murray, eds.), pp. 330–363. S. Karger, Basel.

Palladino, M. A. and Welte, K. (1984). *Ann. NY Acad. Sci.* **437**, 535–539.

Pazin, G. J., Armstrong, J. A. and Lam M. T. (1979). *New Engl. J. Med.* **301**, 225–230.

Penn, L. J. Z. and Williams, B. R. G. (1984). *J. Virol.* **49**, 748–753.

Pollack, M. S., Safai, B., Myskowski, P. L., Gold, J., Pandey, J. and Dupont, B. (1983). *Tissue Antigens* **21**, 1.

Preble, O. T., Black, R. J., Friedman, R. M., Klippel, J. H. and Vilček, J. (1982). *Science* **216**, 429–431.

Preble, O. T., Rook, A. H., Quinnan, G. V., Vilček, J., Friedman, R. M., Steis, R., Gelmann, E. P. and Sonnabend, J. A. (1984). *Ann. NY Acad. Sci.* **437**, 65–75.

Preble, O. T., Rook, A. H., Steis, R., Silverman, R. H., Krause, D., Quinnan, G. V., Masur, H., Jacob, J., Longo, D. and Gelmann, E. P. (1985). *J. Infect. Dis.* **152**, 457–465.

Real, F. X., Oettgen, H. F. and Krown, S. E. (1986a). *J. Clin. Oncol* **4**, 544–551.

Real, F. X., Vadhan-Raj, S., Wong, G., Oettgen, H. F. and Krown, S. E. (1986b). *In* "Proceedings of the 1985 ECCO Symposium on Interferons" (K. Sikora, ed.), in press.

Reddy, M. M., Chinoy, P. Grieco, M. H. (1984). *J. Biol. Resp. Med.* **3**, 379–386.

Reynolds, W. A., Winkelman, R. K. and Soule, E. H. (1965). *Medicine* **44**, 419–443.

Rich, S. A. (1981). *Science* **213**, 772.

Rios, A., Mansell, P. W. A., Newell, G. R., Reuben, J. M., Hersh, E. M. and Gutterman, J. U. (1985a). *J. Clin. Oncol.* **3**, 506–512.

Rios, A., Mansell, P., Newell, G., Reuben, J., Whisnant, J., Hersh, E. M. and Gutterman, J. U. (1985b). *Proc. Amer. Soc. Clin. Oncol.* **4**, 6.

Rook, A. H., Masur, H., Lance, H. C., Frederick, W., Kasahara, T., Macher, A. M., Djeu, J. Y., Manischewitz, J. F., Jackson, L., Fauci, A. S. and Quinnan, G. V. Jr. (1983). *J. Clin. Invest.* **72**, 398–403.

Rook, A. H., Hooks, J. J., Quinnan, G. V. Jr., Lane, H. C., Manischewitz, J. F., Macher, A. M., Masur, H., Fauci, A. S. and Djeu, J. Y. (1985). *J. Immunol.* **134**, 1503–1507.

Rothman, S. (1962). *Acta Un Int Cancer* **18**, 364–371.

Safai, B. and Good, R. A. (1980). *Clin. Bull.* **10**, 62–69.

Safai, B., Miké, V., Giraldo, G., Beth, E. and Good, R. A. (1980). *Cancer* **45**, 1472–1479.

Shaw, G. B., Hahn, B. H., Arya, S. K., Groopman, J. E., Gallo, R. C. and Wong-Stahl, F. (1984). *Science* **226**, 1165–1171.

Siegal, F. P., Lopez, C., Hammer, G. S., Brown, A. E., Kornfeld, S. J., Gold, J., Hassett, J., Hirschman, S. Z., Cunningham-Rundles, S., Adelsberg, B. R., Parham, D. M., Siegal, M., Cunningham-Rundles, C. and Armstrong, D. (1981). *New Engl. J. Med.* **305**, 1439–1444.

Sivak, S. L. and Wormser, G. P. (1985). *New Engl. J. Med.* **313**, 1352.

Skurkovich, S. V. and Eremkina, E. I. (1975). *Ann. Allergy* **35**, 356–360.

Snider, W. D., Simpson, D. M., Aronyk, K. E. and Nielsen, S. L. (1983). *New Engl. J. Med.* **308**, 45.

Taylor, J. F. (1973). *Lancet* **1**, 883–884.

Taylor, J. F. and Ziegler, J. L. (1974). *Br. J. Cancer* **30**, 312–318.

Templeton, A. C. (1981). *Pathol. Annual* 315–336.

Trinchieri, G., Santoli, D., Dee, R. R. and Knowles, B. B. (1978). *J. Exp. Med.* **147**, 1299–1313.

Vadhan-Raj, S., Wong, G., Gnecco, C., Cunningham-Rundles, S., Krim, M., Real, F. X., Oettgen, H. F. and Krown, S. E. (1986a). *Cancer Res.* **46**, 417–425.

Vadhan-Raj, S., Al-Katib, A., Pelus, L., Bhalla, R., Nathan, C. F., Sherwin, S. A., Oettgen, H. F. and Krown, S. E. (1986b). *J. Clin. Oncol.* **4**, 137–146.

Vilček, J. (1982). *In* "Interferon 4" (I. Gresser, ed.), pp. 129–154. Academic Press, London and New York.

Vilček, J. (1984). *Prog. Med. Virol.* **30**, 62–77.

Volberding, P., Valero, R., Rothman, J. and Gee, G. (1984a). *Ann. NY Acad. Sci.* **437**, 439–445.

Volberding, P., Kaslow, K., Bilk, M., Bacchetti, P., Moss, A., Abrams, D., Conant, M. and Ziegler, J. (1984b). *Proc. Amer. Soc. Clin. Oncol.* **3**, 51.

Von Behren, A. and Pesanti, L. (1978). *Amer. Rev. Respir. Dis.* **118**, 1051–1059.

Wallace, J. M., Barbers, R. G., Oishi, J. S., and Prince, H. (1984). *Amer. Rev. Respir. Dis.* **130**, 786–790.

White, D. A., Gellene, R. A., Gupta, S., Cunningham-Rundles, C. and Stover, D. E. (1985). *Chest* **88**, 352–359.

Wing, E. J. and Remington, J. S. (1979). *In* "Principles and Practice of Infectious Diseases" (ed. G. L. Mandell, R. G. Douglas, Jr. and J. E. Bennett, eds.), pp. 83–103. John Wiley, New York.

Yoneda, K. and Walzer, P. D. (1980). *Infect. Immunol.* **29**, 692–703.

Young, K. R. Rankin, J. A., Naegel, G. P., Paul, E. S. and Reynolds, H. Y. (1985). *Ann. Int. Med.* **103**, 522–533.

Ziegler, J., Drew, W. L. and Miner, R. C., (1982). *Lancet* **2**, 000.